therapy is... ★ magic

therapy is... magic

An essential guide to the ups, downs and life-changing experiences of talking therapy

JO LOVE

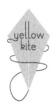

FOR BOO

First published in Great Britain in 2021 by Yellow Kite
An imprint of Hodder & Stoughton
An Hachette UK company

1

Illustrations by Jo Love

The information in this book is not intended to replace or conflict with the advice given to you by your GP or other health professional. All matters regarding your health, including your mental health, should be discussed with your GP. The author and publisher disclaim any liability directly or indirectly from the use of the material in this book by any person.

A CIP catalogue record for this title is available
from the British Library

Hardback ISBN 978 1 529 34843 9
eBook ISBN 978 1 529 34844 6

Typeset in Brandon Grotesque Gothic by Goldust Design

Printed and bound in Great Britain by Clays Ltd, Elcograf S.p.A

Hodder & Stoughton policy is to use papers that are natural, renewable and recyclable products and made from wood grown in sustainable forests. The logging and manufacturing processes are expected to conform to the environmental regulations of the country of origin.

Yellow Kite
Hodder & Stoughton Ltd
Carmelite House
50 Victoria Embankment
London EC4Y 0DZ

www.yellowkitebooks.co.uk

CONTENTS

If you've never sat on a kind-eyed stranger's couch bawling your eyes out as they smile and hand you tissues without judgement or criticism, then you don't know what *magic* you're missing.

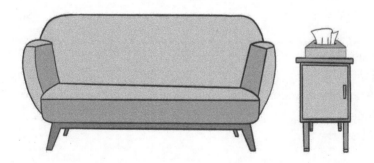

INTRODUCTION

I'm gazing out of my car window at a non-descript suburban street on the London/Essex border in the watery July morning light. The sun is still low and a fragile stillness hangs in the morning air, as if the world is holding its breath in anticipation of the soon-to-come accelerated pace of the day. But my body feels none of this tranquillity; it is on edge. I squeeze my arms and drum my fingers in my lap. My heart rate is higher than it should be and there's a prickling of sweat starting to creep over my skin despite the cool summer morning air coming in from the open window.

My weekly therapy session starts shortly and I'm using these few precious moments beforehand to try to calm the fight or flight reaction fizzing around my body. This isn't a new experience; I've sat in this very spot many times before, silently negotiating with myself. Nevertheless, the trickle of panic about the unknown continues to infuse every cell of my body: 'Oh crap, how on earth am I going to begin to unravel this jumbled muddle of thoughts?' It is as if the volume button of rationality and reason has been turned right down, and instead fear and trepidation scream loudly, 'What if I can't think of anything to say and we just silently stare at each other for the whole session?', 'What if she pushes me too hard?', 'What if I lose control?', 'Oh fuck, what if I cry?' I am overwhelmed. I am lost. But somewhere in this clatter of chaotic thoughts autopilot kicks in – I force myself to get out of the car and approach her door. I make myself ring her doorbell and remind myself to trust in the process.

Fifty minutes later I am walking back to my car transformed. I am untroubled and unburdened by the cacophony of worries that only recently screamed and screeched around my head. I am liberated with relief. But how can it be that in this short window of time I feel both emotionally and physically lighter? I can viscerally feel the weight lifted from my shoulders. It's as if my therapist has gently twisted open a pressure valve somewhere deep inside me, allowing the stress to be released with control and a calm clarity to fill the space left behind. I feel listened to, understood and emotionally held. Therapy is magic.

Don't get me wrong, therapy can also be uncomfortable, confronting and often exhausting, and I can leave feeling anything but 'light'. But, this doesn't stop therapy feeling magical, as it's often in those hard sessions when something deep is unlocked and the magic truly lives. Changes start to happen and the pain turns into gain. It's very normal, and likely a positive sign you're making real progress, if you don't enjoy therapy all of the time.

I'm Jo. I'm 37 years old. I have a great husband and a beautiful daughter, who makes me proud every day. I studied and practised law for many years at one of the world's premier law firms. I have an undeniably privileged and comfortable life and, as a white, privately-schooled, university-educated, heterosexual, cisgender woman in the UK, my experiences, by many objective measures, have been easy.

I say this not to incite envy and give you reason to stop reading (to be fair, I wouldn't blame you if you did), but because first and foremost I think it is important that I am upfront about my privilege as it will undoubtedly have had an impact, not on my mental health as such, but certainly on my treatment and the support I have received. Secondly, because to read that last paragraph and to look at my life from the outside, you'd never guess that I struggle every day with my self-esteem, my self-worth and my value, not only as a mother and a friend, but as a human being. You wouldn't know that I regularly drift in and out of periods of mental ill health that can be both disabling and alarming (for myself and those around me), despite the regularity with which they appear in my life. And, of course, even when the cloak of mental illness descends, I can normally hide it well. Most of the time. I function, most of the time. I wear the mask of being 'OK', most of the time.

What does someone with a mental health condition look like anyway? In my experience it certainly isn't how 'mad' people are stereotypically represented in the movies or on TV. The mentally ill are often portrayed as mumbling, erratic, incompetent, dangerous, chaotic, slovenly and undeserving, which only serves to distance 'them' from the rest of 'us', perpetuating fear and ignorance. Despite having mental health conditions from a relatively young age, my mental health knowledge, prejudice and language were severely lacking for an embarrassingly long time. My internal cringe-o-meter shoots off the scale when I think about all the times I stereotypically labelled others and myself. I'd even jokingly describe myself as being 'a little bit OCD' long before, in a cruel twist of irony, years later I would in fact be diagnosed with dermatillomania, (chronic skin-picking), which, it turns out, is in the OCD family.

For many people with mental health conditions like myself, we often appear 'normal', whatever that might be. We are often fully contributing members of society on the surface, but underneath there's a much darker and more complex story going on. I've long used my social media channels to highlight the disparity between what is happening on the surface and what is actually going on beneath, through a campaign called #DepressionWearsLippy.

It gained traction a few years ago and globally thousands of women (and a few men and pets too) have shared their lipstick selfies, and many more have used the hashtag since, showing that mental illness doesn't have to look a specific way. The idea came about a couple of years ago after an online troll accused me of fabricating my condition, saying that I looked too groomed to suffer anxiety or depression. My response was to show the world that as often as mental health conditions hide away or look the way we expect, mental health issues are also all around us and look like every one of us. Sometimes they wear lipstick and sometimes they do not. Mental health issues cross all social constructs, genders and ethnicities; they affect the rich, poor, old and young. Having a mental health condition is not a choice and they don't discriminate with who they affect, so neither should we in our behaviour towards people who have them.

Therapy has been my lifeline; it has changed my life in a way I could never have anticipated. At the time of writing, I have seen a therapist or been in therapy at various points for roughly half of my life. That's over 18 years of spilling my innermost thoughts to numerous strangers for bouts of various talking therapies for multiple reasons. If this were a marriage, it'd be our porcelain anniversary – a material known for both its toughness and also its fragility. Which I think is fitting, considering the context. And without wanting to bore you senseless with a long list of diagnoses, I think it's important to let you know that at different points in my life my therapy has been for anxiety, depression, postnatal depression, post-traumatic stress disorder, compulsive and intrusive thoughts and behaviours, as well as other things that have fallen short of a clear categorisation, and now it's more about my mental wellness, self-esteem, self-improvement and self-care.

A quick aside: it's important to remember that, for some,

diagnoses can be helpful in validating their suffering and giving them a platform from which to speak about distress and access help. However, this isn't always the case. Some diagnoses can have the opposite effect, feeling stigmatising and leading to negative evaluations by the public, family members and even the person with mental health concerns themselves.

EIGHT LIES I'VE TOLD MYSELF ABOUT MY MENTAL ILLNESS DIAGNOSIS

1 'I have failed; I should have been able to control my mood myself.'
2 'I am weak. I have brought this upon myself.'
3 'This means I am crazy.'
4 'This means I am a fundamentally flawed human.'
5 'My life is over.'
6 'I will never amount to anything.'
7 'I will never have friends.'
8 'I may as well give up.'

I do not claim to understand how the magic of therapy works; all I know is that something incredible happens when you find another human you can open up to and they are trained to listen and support you in response. I think it's probably quite important I say at the outset that, as far as I am aware, NO ACTUAL MAGIC is involved in therapy, despite at times me being utterly convinced that some kind of sorcery is at play in my therapist's office. But what is unquestionably true for me is that it has felt as though something magical happens in therapy and this book seeks to lift the veil on a secretive and sadly still stigmatised world.

I also feel compelled to let you know that there is no magic pill, no quick fix, no incantation or spell to cast. Therapy is hard. It's hard to get the courage to go to therapy; it's hard to find the right person who makes you feel safe, held and comfortable; it's hard to trust the process when progress is slow; it's hard when you doubt yourself; and it's hard when you come away feeling worse than when you went in. Even when it's great, you have a therapist you connect with and you're making good progress, it's still bloody hard work. Worth it, every second, but hard.

To continue in arse-covering mode, I want to warn you that this book touches on many triggering subjects, including self-harm and suicide. If this means it's not for you, I'm sad to see you go, but I quite understand. I also want you to know that I'm speaking from my personal experiences with therapy and mental illness. If you or someone you know may be living with mental illness or mental health issues, please talk to a qualified medical professional or encourage them to, because I am not a doctor, nor am I qualified as a therapist.

There is so much that is kept hidden when it comes to mental health, so much that happens behind closed doors, so much that we keep locked away from the world and often even from ourselves. In this book I throw those doors wide open and tackle

MYTHS ABOUT THERAPY

Myth: 'I don't need a therapist. I'm smart enough to solve my own problems.'
Truth: We all have our blind spots. Intelligence has nothing to do with whether or not we'd benefit from therapy. A good therapist doesn't tell you what to do or how to live your life. They will give you an experienced outside perspective and help you gain insight into yourself so you can make better choices.

Myth: 'Therapy is for crazy people.'
Truth: Therapy is for people who have enough self-awareness to realise they need a helping hand, whether that is to help them cope with a mental illness or issue, or simply because they wish to learn tools and techniques to help their lives, for example to become more self-confident or emotionally balanced.

Myth: 'All therapists want to talk about is my parents and childhood.'
Truth: While exploring family relationships can sometimes clarify our thoughts and behaviours later in life, that is not the sole focus of therapy and, depending on the type of therapy you have, might feature very seldomly, if at all. The primary focus of pretty much all therapy is on what you need to change – unhealthy patterns and symptoms in your life. Therapy really is not about blaming your parents or dwelling for too long on the past.

many of the less spoken about aspects of mental health and how to access support. So, despite my dad telling me to never talk publicly about money, politics or religion, I think this book would be doing a disservice to you the reader but also to myself if it didn't address at least the first two of these to some degree. I really don't think we can, nor should we try to, separate mental health support in any of its forms from less palatable topics such as politics, finance, social issues and race because, to me, they are inextricably intertwined. Our lives don't operate in a vacuum and neither does our mental health and by extension therapy. Not to mention that much emotional distress is often caused by many of these exact issues.

I've realised a lot of things through trial and error that I wish someone had told me before I ventured into the secretive and often entirely misunderstood world of therapy. I've also come to a place in my life where I strongly feel if we are open and honest with our truths and share our vulnerabilities, not only can we help others, but also real change will happen.

These pages contain the very comfort and reassurance I have craved over the years in therapy from the perspective of someone actually doing the work, learning the lessons and making the mistakes. This book doesn't just lift the lid on the incredible, unique conversation and relationship that happens between the therapist and the client, it throws that box wide open to give you a real flavour of what therapy feels like from the rarely heard client perspective. We shall begin with what I wish I had known before this all began...

▶ I shouldn't wear mascara to my therapy sessions.

▶ I will never lie on a couch during therapy.

▶ No one will ever say, 'So how does that make you feel?'

- My therapist is NOT a mind reader.
- Going to therapy doesn't make me weak.
- Therapy will be awkward.
- Therapy will be hard.
- Therapy will change my life.
- Therapy saved my life.
- Therapy is NOT bullshit.
- Therapy is magic.

From the Other Chair
THERAPY

Throughout the book you will see pop-outs like this from the professionals when something needs a little deeper explanation or the ex-lawyer in me has sensed this is something I'm vastly underqualified to be explaining. So for our first quick word from the 'other chair', I want to draw your attention to the fact that I am going to be using the term 'therapy' throughout this book rather loosely to mean all forms of talking therapy unless I specifically say otherwise. Talking therapy encapsulates a number of things, so this is as good a moment as any to bring in the big guns and let them guide us.

As Dr Emma Svanberg, clinical psychologist (aka @mumologist on Instagram), explains, therapy can refer to various treatments. All involve talking to another human being who is a trained professional about your current difficulties, what may be causing them and the paths available to make a change.

There are many different types of talking therapy, but they all aim to:

▶ give you a safe time and place to talk to someone who won't judge you

▶ help you make sense of things and understand yourself better

▶ help you resolve complicated feelings or find ways to reach acceptance

▶ help you recognise unhelpful patterns in the way you think or act, and find ways to change them (if you want to)

▶ experience a relationship with someone who is there to think only about you

Throughout the book you will see reference made to 'therapy', but you might also hear people talking about:

▶ counselling

▶ talking therapy

▶ psychotherapy

▶ psychological therapy

▶ talking treatment

These refer to the different training undergone by therapists. There is overlap in the methods used by therapists, but there are different training requirements for different types of therapists.

Confusingly, you might hear people generically refer to therapy that they have had as 'counselling'. Often these are interchangeable terms, but very roughly sessions with a counsellor are usually shorter term, whereas a psychotherapist will typically see you over the longer term.

Unlike other mental health professionals, such as psychologists and counsellors, psychiatrists must be medically qualified doctors who have chosen to specialise in psychiatry. This means they can prescribe medication as well as recommend other forms of treatment. Most psychiatrists work as part of community mental health teams, in outpatient clinics or on hospital wards. We'll discuss the different types of therapy in more detail in Chapter Ten (see page 185).

Maybe right now therapy feels really scary or it's something you aren't able to connect with. Maybe you're unsure where to start or just don't know whether therapy is right for you. Maybe your family or friends are pressurising you to see someone and you're apprehensive. Or maybe you know someone in therapy and you want to know how to best support them. Perhaps you're curious about what the potential benefits might be or how it all actually works. Possibly you're in therapy, but are finding it hard going, unsure of whether to give up or stick at it. Maybe you are in therapy and are looking for tips on how to get the most from it or want to know how to end it in the least awkward way possible.

Whether you're a lifelong therapy-goer or a complete newbie, you can use this book as a guide to bettering your sessions and, ultimately, the way that you feel. Whatever the reason, come on in – you're in the right place.

The book is split into two parts. Part One is a series of my real-life experiences and mental health lows that found me winding up on the proverbial couch as well as many of the lessons I have learned from sitting my butt down over and over again on said couch. Part Two is also filled with many examples from my own experiences in the client chair to help you better understand what it is you're getting into and give you a realistic insight into what can happen, but I also share all my tips and strategies that have helped me over the years to make the most of my experience inside the therapy room and my mental wellness on the outside.

Therefore, whether you're looking for more information about therapy, help with breaking out of seemingly endless cycles of burnout, tips on how to curb your perfectionism, advice on how to say no, or you'd like some pointers on dealing with anxiety, grief, depression and everything in between, this book is most definitely for you.

Above all else, I hope that reading this book will help you to talk more comfortably about these very normal struggles, whether that is to a therapist, a friend or just to yourself.

Therapy thoughts

'Therapy is not as scary as I first thought! I was so terrified to sit in front of someone, look them in the eye, and talk about the deepest, darkest parts of myself. I wish I had known how much of a release it would be!'
Jonny Benjamin MBE, award-winning mental health campaigner, film producer, public speaker and author of *The Stranger on the Bridge*

Part One
THERAPY IS...

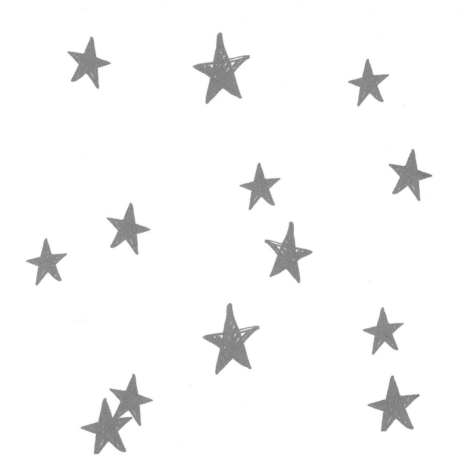

Chapter One
THERAPY IS
Uncomfortable

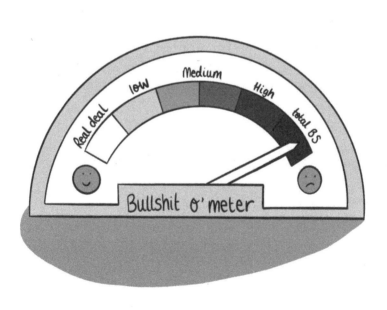

Before I experienced it, I used to think therapy was a load of bullshit. Which then sadly my experiences with my first few rather appalling therapists did nothing to soften. I could see no value whatsoever in sitting and dissecting my past decisions and events ad nauseam, trying to figure out exactly what had gone 'wrong' just so some patronising bore could then not really 'fix' anything but instead ask me to talk about it again and again.

However, I could see that therapy had its place; in my opinion, it was reserved for those with the most serious mental health afflictions only. For everyone else who had therapy, I believed they did so through a thin-skinned narcissistic pursuit of approval. It was for the weak. It was for the feeble. The whiners. The whingers. To my mind, all this talking, all this 'gut-spewing nonsense', was a load of hot air and often just a great moneymaking scam for the therapists. As you can probably tell, I viewed those who went to 'see someone' with a heavy dose of disdain, I sneered at their seemingly ludicrous outpouring of emotion. I'm embarrassed and ashamed to admit it now, but, deep down, I thought myself superior to what I saw as their lack of resilience. Looking back, my ignorance would be laughable if it wasn't so pitiful itself. I was insulted by their failure to embody the British stiff upper lip that my parents, having themselves been raised by a generation who had 'survived the war', had instilled in me. I heard loud and clear the message not to 'make a fuss' and acted accordingly. Therefore, any opening up and sharing of one's problems publicly was simply unacceptable. Consequently, I learned to be an expert bottler and brave face putter-on-er. I wasn't just in denial; I worshiped at the altar of it. But then one chance encounter changed all that.

MY MASK BEGINS TO SLIP

'You're batshit crazy; you need your head looked at. No, seriously, you need to see someone...'

I'm in shock; the words are disdainfully spat at me, packed full of scorn and derision. They seem suspended between us, hanging awkwardly in the air. I've heard them, but I haven't really taken them in – it's like the sound waves have physically hit my ears but the meaning hasn't yet reached my mind. My thoughts start racing. I must have misheard, he must have been talking to someone else – but no he is definitely looking at me and he is most certainly talking to me. Then BAM they hit me – the words are suddenly in me, unravelling me, spreading their poison almost instantly with a thousand tiny daggers delivering their venomous sting.

I am 18, newly at law school. It's 2am and I am standing in the rain outside a grim Birmingham nightclub where I have without doubt consumed more unnaturally neon-coloured alcopops than I should have done. I'm arguing with a boy whose name I no longer remember, over some minor indiscretion that I can now no longer recall. As I type these words, I've sat for a few moments contemplating what might have led up to this moment of drunk fury in the infamously damp Midlands drizzle, but the truth is that the passage of time, like the rain, has simply washed the details away.

However, the raw stinging memory of the words still vividly remains all these years later. A tiny distant echo of their powerful punch still lives on inside me even now, when the girl who heard them is so drastically different from the woman who sits here today talking to you. The force of the condemnation remains and what I felt in that moment as those words landed their thunderous blows was 'I am a massive failure'. The secret I'd been carrying around had been exposed. The mask I'd been wearing had slipped. I had been seen. Really seen. I was crushed; I had spent my entire life trying not to be seen.

At first look I don't seem like someone who doesn't want to be seen. I seem pretty confident, I'm slim, I'm reasonably clever and I know it. I'm opinionated and, in the past, I have certainly used my looks to my advantage. But I am also an introvert, I struggle with my self-worth, confidence and sense of identity. I am a people-pleaser, a chameleon changing with my environment and who I am talking to, making sure I am fitting in, blending in. I shape-shift so often that I'm regularly left unpicking a tangled knot of unknown identities. I am a perfectionist. And something I have learned through many years of therapy is that perfectionists are often this way because we want to blend in rather than stand out. Somewhere along the way we've developed this coping mechanism to keep us safe, as we are afraid that the world is going to see us for who we really are and in that moment we won't measure up, we won't be liked, we will have failed.

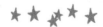

Those toxic little words uttered by a drunken long-forgotten boy on a dark street stayed with me far longer than the next day's hangover; they seeped in and replayed repeatedly, burrowing into me like a parasite slowly worming its way through my flesh into my body. Maybe I *was* crazy. Maybe I *did* need to see someone. I was definitely a failure – that I was sure of. But I was OK, wasn't I? Everyone is a little bit low at times, right? I was going out, I had friends, I looked happy. But I couldn't shake the sadness, the feeling that I was spinning out of control. It was taking all my effort and energy to keep myself steady, to keep looking normal. But the spin proved impossible to contain, its unstoppable force churned through me. I was self-harming – I would bite the tiny

JO'S TOOLKIT: TEN SIGNS YOU MIGHT BE A PERFECTIONIST

1 Your sense of self-worth often hangs on others' approval or your accomplishments.

2 It's hard to recognise or celebrate your successes because nothing you do ever feels quite good enough.

3 Your failure or mistakes feel like the proof you need of your inadequacy and are very difficult to forget.

4 You find it hard to delegate and trust others to do things properly.

5 Criticism can totally crush you.

6 You have high expectations not just of yourself but of others too.

7 You have a tendency to procrastinate or avoid doing something altogether if you don't think you'll be able to do it perfectly.

8 You spend a lot of time and energy masking your flaws.

9 You link being perfect with being liked.

10 You find yourself focusing on the end product of a task rather than the process of learning or enjoying the doing.

hard plastic bobbles off the end of a hairgrip with my teeth and dig it deep into places no one could see, but as time went on these were becoming more noticeable and I would need to hurt more to feel the same release of pressure. This wasn't normal, I wasn't coping and now people around me had started to notice.

I tried to push the comment away, ignore it and carry on. But it was as if a chain reaction had begun in my mind and hundreds of tiny fires of self-loathing ignited into a roaring inferno of depression. I felt on the verge of implosion. And so, only a few days later, I found myself where many of my therapy journeys over the years would begin – weeping, or more accurately hyperventilating, and enormously oversharing to a hassled and slightly irritated-looking GP.

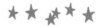

I remember being too afraid to use my university's free counselling service as it was linked to the University Advice Centre, which was located right in the epicentre of our Students' Union. Not only was the Advice Centre in the beating heart of my social

NEED HELP NOW?

If you are reading this and are looking for help now, please skip ahead to page 260 as there I share some of the brilliant mental health resources – including crisis resources – I have come across in my time, both online and offline. Chapter Ten also lists the various ways you can access therapy in the UK, both privately and through the NHS, as well as other lesser known routes.

life, the desk was manned by students, giving it 100 per cent certainty in my mind that I would be outed in my quest for help if I went down this route. This could not happen. It was bad enough that I had been exposed by one person; I couldn't have anyone else know I was 'batshit'.

Ironically, the day before the GP visit was the first time I had my first full-blown panic attack, although I didn't understand what it was at the time. Looking back, it's pretty easy to join the dots; however, I couldn't see then how close to the edge of the cliff I was standing, and how the topple had been inevitable.

I was sitting at my desk in my university room when, out of nowhere, my heart started thumping very loudly, too loudly. It felt like the blood was passing through my ears with a loud rhythmic thump, thump, thump; this was not right. It was like when you're a kid and hang upside down for too long on the monkey bars – all the blood rushing and swimming around your brain – except I hadn't been hanging upside down. I had been sitting doing nothing very remarkable. My chest was tight, too tight, it felt like I was choking. Suddenly, I was hot and sticky, so much so that I went to run my face under cold water. But as I stood up to go to the sink, a sudden trembling travelled down my body from my hands into my arms and legs, leaving me unsteady on my feet. My heart seemed to pound even faster, even harder. I couldn't breathe. I felt like I was being held underwater with no way of coming up for air. I tried taking a deep breath to calm myself, but my breaths were sharp and shallow, and my body seemed to have other ideas as I struggled to get the smallest amount of air into my lungs. My body and mind were not my own. My vision got darker and narrower and felt kaleidoscopic, a little bit like when you close your eyes and press down on your eyelids to 'see stars'.

But again, I wasn't closing my eyes or pushing anything. The sense of dread and fear pulsed through me; 'Something's wrong,

JO'S TOOLKIT: FOUR WEIRD TIPS THAT HAVE HELPED ME WITH PANIC ATTACKS

1   *Counting*. Recently I found that trying to focus on something else, such as counting numbers out of order, seems to work, I think because it requires a certain level of concentration. You could try counting the numbers one to nine out of order or something like taking sevens or threes from one hundred as many times as possible. Or for me, just attempting my eight times table tends to work!

2   *Going upside down*. Literally, I lie over the edge of a sofa, bench, chair, whatever, and just breathe. I think the different perspective helps me remember to breathe and focus only on the things I can see around me.

3   *Grounding*. I look around to find five things I can see, four things I can touch, three things I can hear, two things I can smell and one thing I can taste. This often helps when I feel like I have lost control of my surroundings.

4   *Water*. I've found sometimes that if I run cold water over the inside of my wrist it helps.

something's wrong, something's wrong', which was quickly replaced with, 'You're dying' and 'This is what death feels like, you're going to die here and now.'

Eventually, I slowly sank to the floor. I don't know how long the whole thing lasted or how much time passed before I was able to get up and steady myself; it honestly could have been 30 seconds or an hour. What I do know is that I crawled from the floor to the bed, my brain feeling like it had been splintered in two, and slept for 13 hours straight, quite literally as though the life had been drained right out of me.

I told no one about this. Not even those closest to me at the time. And although these attacks would be increasingly familiar to me, this is the way it stayed for another 17 years.

From the Other Chair
PANIC ATTACKS

As Dr Sophie Mort, clinical psychologist (aka @_drsoph on Instagram), explains, a panic attack is a type of fear-based bodily response. Panic attacks usually come on very quickly, sometimes with an obvious trigger, like getting stuck in a lift for example, but other times for no apparent reason. Symptoms vary from person to person, but include experiences such as a sudden surge of fear, tightness in the chest, a racing heartbeat or palpitations, sweating, shaking, chest pain, feeling like it is hard to breathe or feeling dizzy, faint or light-headed, or disconnected from your body.

Most panic attacks last for between 5 and 20 minutes, though sometimes they can last longer. And although they are usually short in nature, during that time the feelings can be highly distressing, with some people reporting feelings of losing control or terror, or feeling faint or worried they are having a heart attack or dying.

Some people have attacks once or twice in their life, while others have them several times a week. Although panic attacks can be very frightening, they're not dangerous. And, people who experience panic attacks respond very well to therapeutic treatment, such as cognitive behavioural therapy (CBT), where they are taught grounding techniques and breathing exercises that can de-escalate anxiety, and often stop a panic attack in its tracks (see page 188 for more on CBT).

After happily chatting to my GP about an entirely fictional ear pain for a good five minutes and hearing the words, 'Is there anything else I can help with today?', something rather strange started to happen. I remember thinking 'It's now or never' and at that very moment I could hear myself speaking, but I felt displaced somehow. Not an out-of-body experience by a long shot, but it certainly felt as though my autopilot had kicked in and my mouth was speaking but my mind wasn't fully in the room. And despite having had the very clear intention to keep things 'light' and breezy, for reasons that are still somewhat foggy to me, I decided in that moment to open the emotional floodgates to this unsuspecting stranger. It all came out: my self-harming, self-loathing, lack of self-confidence, mood swings and depression.

Needless to say, I proceeded to spend the next 45 minutes of the strict 10-minute time slot making inconsolable, unrecognisable noises and emptying her tissue box to such an extent that my sleeve was then required to step up to the plate.

I had imploded. Eventually, she was able to prise me out of her office and I was sent away with a puffy face, a prescription for medication and a referral for talking therapy.

Medication. Therapy. It was all too much.

I stuffed the prescription into the first bin I saw. I can still recall the defiance and fury as I did it like it was yesterday. I told myself pills were for lunatics and they would make me a zombie. I thought many negative things about myself at this point in time, but I was fairly confident that a lunatic I was not, and a zombie didn't sound all that fun either.

The therapy part proved harder to ignore. There was nothing to stuff in a bin and I now appeared to be 'in the system', as they say. Meaning I was regularly receiving very official-looking letters on headed paper with 'Mental Health NHS Foundation Trust' written on them. I won't beat about the bush – this freaked me the fuck out. The shame I felt each time I received a letter crushed me. Each one proved to me my failure right there in black and white. I had never heard the words 'mental health' in any other way than in an extremely negative context and therefore seeing those words used on correspondence addressed to me was almost too much to bear. I had failed before I had even begun. I was certain that if anyone found out about this they would think I was crazy and unstable, and needed to be locked up. I worried about what impact it might have on my legal career. I'd like to go back in time and tell myself I hadn't failed as a human by 'going to see someone'. It was not a stain on my identity; it was simply a matter of being human.

My very first step on the therapy ladder was strange and unquestionably harrowing. My GP had referred me to a psychiatrist who would decide what my treatment would look like, including managing my medication and monitoring my progress.

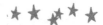

As I walk to my first appointment with the psychiatrist, my insides feel like they are filled with stones; with every step my breakfast is threatening to make a reappearance. I arrive at the single-storey unremarkable brick building that at first glance looks a little like it could be a care home for the elderly. I can't seem to find the way in. I pace the perimeter feeling increasingly panicked as no obvious entrance or reception materialises and my appointment time ticks ever closer. Finally, I find a door with an intercom speaker panel and stutter into it that I am here for an appointment. I hear the system buzz and the door clicks open. I quickly hurry inside, the door locking shut behind me. An irrational thought flits through my mind that I will be locked in forever unable to get out, wrongly mistaken for a mad person and not believed when I plead sanity. I find my pace quickening. I bolt through the maze-like identical corridors panicked and terrified of what I might glimpse behind the locked doors.

Eventually I arrive in the waiting room sweating, my heart stumbling over its own rhythm. As I sit there surrounded by other people, I am surprised, but enormously relieved, to discover that they all look completely 'normal'. Eventually, a man appears and calls my name. He is a nicely dressed, bespectacled West African man who looks to be around 50 or so. He has a kind face and a soft voice.

As I follow him through some heavy double doors and into his office beyond, he asks if I mind a student sitting in the room with us, explaining how they will only observe and how it helps with their training. I mumble that this is fine, but as I enter his office behind him I realise this is anything but fine. Sat in the corner of his office, which looks very much like any ordinary doctor's office, is the medical student. But it's not any old med student, it's someone I know. Of course it is. And I don't just know him vaguely. Oh no, this is someone I really know. He's part of my inner friendship circle, dating my good friend. In fact, I'd been having drinks with him only the night before and I would awkwardly find myself avoiding eye contact over a pub table a few short days later.

Oh the shame.

We lock eyes and both flush with embarrassment. He mumbles that he should step out of the room and I nod, lowering my mortified gaze.

I fumble through the appointment as my insides are on fire in humiliation. After what feels like an excruciating eternity, I leave the psychiatrist's office with a severely bruised pride, a diagnosis of generalised anxiety disorder (GAD) and depression, and a recommendation to see a therapist for a course of CBT.

From the Other Chair
GENERALISED ANXIETY DISORDER and DEPRESSION

As Dr Mayowa Aina, clinical psychologist (aka @dr.mayus on Instagram), explains, generalised anxiety disorder (GAD) is a diagnosis that can be made when you experience regular or uncontrollable worries about many different things in your everyday life. It is normal to feel anxious sometimes, especially at times when your life is stressful. However, if your worries and fears are hard to control, distressing or so constant that they interfere with your ability to function and relax day to day, you may be experiencing symptoms of GAD.

GAD is a common anxiety disorder that involves constant

and chronic worrying, nervousness and tension. Unlike a phobia, where your fear can be connected to a specific thing or situation, the anxiety of GAD is hard to pin down to a specific trigger. Instead, many people describe a general feeling of dread or unease that seems to colour their whole life. There are lots of different symptoms of chronic worry and so GAD can be quite a broad diagnosis, meaning that the problems you experience with GAD might be quite different from another person's. In addition, chronic worrying is often a maintaining factor in mental health difficulties and so GAD often presents itself with other mental health concerns.

Depression is a very common mental concern affecting more than 264 million people worldwide. It is more than simply feeling a bit fed up or unhappy for a few days. It affects different people in different ways, but it can show itself as persistent sadness and a lack of interest or pleasure in previously rewarding or enjoyable activities that goes on for a few weeks or months rather than days. Depression can also disturb sleep and appetite; tiredness and poor concentration are common. The effects of depression can range from mild to severe. The symptoms can be long-lasting or recurrent and can dramatically affect a person's ability to function and live a rewarding life.

Sometimes, there is an obvious cause of depression, such as a life-changing event like losing your job or experiencing a bereavement, and at other times depression can seem to come on out of the blue.

Regardless of whether you can identify a cause or not, depression is often an understandable response to unmanageable and distressing life events.

JO'S TOOLKIT: FIVE THINGS NOT TO SAY TO SOMEONE WITH DEPRESSION

1   'But you have such a great life!'

2   'We all get a bit down sometimes; you just need to look on the bright side.'

3   'Have you tried yoga/meditation/mindfulness/ CBD oil?'

4   'Oh, I don't believe in mental illness.'

5   'But you don't seem depressed to me!'

THERAPY IS BULLSHIT

'What's that smell?' It's all I can think of. The stench hits me in jarringly warm waves of air with a somehow familiar, funky, ripe, organic whiff.

This is my first-ever session, with my first-ever therapist and I know that I should be concentrating, but I can't. In these initial moments, as my eyes wildly search for the pungent source of the smell, they don't see the condensation-filled windows with their insidious green-black mould creeping around their edges spreading on to the neighbouring windowsills, the dank grey-green walls that have ancient blobs of Blu-Tack still attached to them and ghost outlines of long since removed pieces of paper. I don't notice how uncomfortable the once red, now faded to orange, plastic stackable school-style chair I'm sat on is. My brain bypasses the unidentifiable stains on the same brown, bobbly woolly jumper that would repeatedly sit in front of me for weeks on end. These specifics pass me by as I sit in that room for the first time, but are details that later I will fixate upon, staring at them minute after minute, week after week, for hours and hours.

Back to the stench that now is so powerful I feel like I may pass out. I have it – I've finally located its source. There, just behind the slightly dishevelled figure in front of me, sits a pair of ancient, grubby-looking walking boots that are propped up in front of an old electric heater that doesn't look like it has ever passed any sort of electrical safety test, which is rhythmically blasting the mucky boots' warm, overripe Camembert smell into the room.

Uh oh, this is not going to work. At this point the therapist has barely even opened his beard-covered halitosis-infused mouth, but I know in that very first moment that this is absolutely, most definitely, without a shadow of a doubt, not going to work.

Sadly, he doesn't do anything to make up for this piss-poor start to my therapeutic journey. I can unhappily report that the foul odour of the room sadly never decreases from that first day, the filthy boots are a regular fixture, and the stench is frequently added to with his brazen belches (and occasionally the far from subtle breaking of wind).

His technique also leaves a lot to be desired. Every week he begins by asking me how things have been that previous week, and he proceeds to pick out a seemingly arbitrary detail from what I have said and then we spend an infuriatingly long time poring over it in detail. He also seems completely preoccupied with a rather bizarre 'game' that he's concocted where he constantly tries to pinpoint geographically exactly where my accent is from but I'm not allowed to tell him until he has guessed it correctly (for the reader who may have never heard my not-so-dulcet voice, it's very unremarkable; some might deem it 'posh southerner', but I would say it has a rather 'bland middle-class' intonation with no discernible hint of geographic origin). This game means that, rather distractingly, my dialogue is regularly punctuated with loud interruptions of 'Henley?', 'St Albans!', 'Norwich!!?' Even with my very limited knowledge of what therapy would entail, I don't think this should be it.

As if this wasn't enough, he never seems to recall very much about the things we have discussed previously. It is like each session is the first, meaning we never actually move forward to doing any kind of real work. This is supposed to be CBT (a fairly interactive, practical form of therapy by all accounts – see page 188 for more info), but I just turn up, talk for 50 minutes about an innocuous part of my week, while staring at the wall and the mould-infested windows, fidget uncomfortably in my plastic chair, do my best to ignore the foul odour and then leave feeling no better and usually quite a bit worse.

Unsurprisingly, I run out of steam for the sessions after a few months and he agrees with me at that point that we haven't really made any progress at all and we should probably part ways. The only tangible advice I can ever recall him giving is saying, 'Have you considered joining an amateur dramatics society?', which makes me think that at best he is calling me a drama queen, and at worst he hasn't believed a single word I have said.

Therapy is most definitely bullshit.

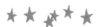

As bleak as this experience of my first therapist sounds, I want to hold my hands up and acknowledge that, looking back, it's clear to me I also played a pivotal role in this dismal dalliance. As objectively terrible as he was, I can see now, with the 20/20

JO'S TOOLKIT: TWELVE WARNING SIGNS TO WATCH OUT FOR

Your therapist...

1   ...falls asleep during your session

2   ...forgets your name (or other important details)

3   ...shares too much of their own life with you

4   ...smells bad

5   ...hits on you or makes inappropriate comments

6   ...rolls their eyes or fidgets

7   ...compulsively clicks a pen

8   ...picks their teeth/nose

9   ...seems distracted or preoccupied

10   ...is rude

11   ...makes you feel uncomfortable

12   ...listens but doesn't hear

vision that only hindsight allows, that I wasn't open, I wasn't ready. I hadn't found the right therapy or the right therapist and I needed to deal with my own internal stigma, as well as that of those around me, before this would eventually change. I wanted help in theory, but not actually in practice. I was afraid to open up; afraid to voice my hurt; afraid I'd be analysed; afraid I'd be seen. Whoever I had met, however nurturing and safe the experience may have been, I think I wasn't ready to be seen by others and especially not by myself. Therapy is magic, but you need to be ready, open and want to work on you.

Therapy thoughts

Hope Virgo, leading eating disorder campaigner and author, tells me that her worst therapy moment was *'when a therapist told me to eat a pizza and feel rubbish and then it would be OK. My face must have said it all. I got through the rest of the session like an adolescent bratty teenager and then never went again.'*

Chapter Two
THERAPY IS
Awkward

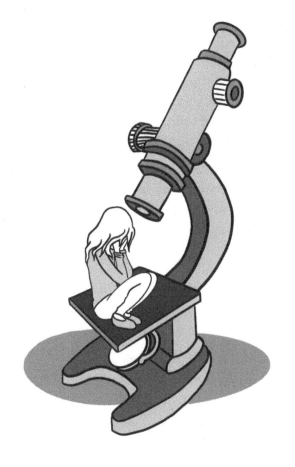

What are the rules here anyway?

Why are they just looking at me; why aren't they speaking?

What do they want me to do?

Is this the way all therapy sessions start? Surely not.

OK, OK, I can do this. Think. What do they want me to say? Probably something about my feelings, but I can't just launch into that can I?

Maybe I should ask them what they want me to say? No... that doesn't feel right.

Perhaps I should ask them how they are. That's what polite strangers do. No, that's not right either – I don't think you're supposed to spend therapy doing small talk. Oh God, I'm such a fuck up, I can't even do this right!

What happens if I don't say anything? Will they just sit and stare at me for the entire 50 minutes? Surely not. Surely not?!

Why can't someone tell me what the hell I am meant to do?

Why haven't I said anything yet? This silence is unbearable.

What the hell is wrong with me?!

Gah, this is so awkward!

After 18 years of therapy, I've had some great moments, but I've also had some toe-curlingly, 'ground open up and swallow me now', embarrassingly awkward moments too. Because, let's face it, therapy can be really bloody awkward. It's awkward to sit in a small room staring at a stranger not knowing how to fill the empty air. It's awkward to be vulnerable; it's awkward to admit you need help; it's awkward to face uncomfortable truths; it's awkward to open up and let another person see all the things you keep so well hidden from the world. Not to mention all the ugly crying and snot a therapist has to witness!

When writing this book, I decided to pick the hive mind and ask my followers on Instagram what their most awkward therapy moments have been, and here's what they said:

- Bedroom chat, especially if the therapist is of the opposite sex (one follower even said hers reminds her too much of her dad so sex cannot be discussed – ever).

- Fancying your therapist.

- Being flirted with by your therapist (being flirted with as a therapist).

- Not knowing how to end the therapeutic relationship (help on this later in the book).

- Wanting to initiate a hug but fearing rejection.

- Having your therapist turn up to your session in fancy dress (a bright pink seventies outfit apparently!).

- Your therapist mishearing your name, which you are then too polite to correct them on, and having to go with the 'new' name for a good few years.

- Your therapist falling asleep on you.

- Not eating beforehand and getting a loud rumbling tummy.

- Forgetting to pay (this happens surprisingly often to me in fact).

- Crying for the first time in front of them.

- Non-stop crying, followed by apologising for crying, followed by apologising for apologising, followed by more crying.

- Snorting while crying.

- Accidentally farting when crying or sneezing.

- And finally, one story involving a malfunctioning catheter, which is probably a little too intimate to share here, but trust me when I tell you, it sounded awkward as hell!

MY WORLD SPLITS IN TWO

It is late February and the long, dark, cold days of winter are starting to loosen their vice-like grip on the world. The weak winter light is almost imperceptibly beginning to give way to something more vibrant. The tiny buds of green on the trees feel like small symbols of hope.

I can feel my own annual hibernation beginning to end too. The pieces of myself that every year I painstakingly and meticulously tuck away and switch off during the winter months, much like the trees turning into echoes of their summer vibrancy in order to survive, are starting to slowly unfurl and come back to life. I am shedding my coat of winter melancholy and gloom, tentatively exposing my pale limbs to the new season.

Yet, as the fizz of promise and hope hangs almost tangibly in the air, my world is about to crash down, forever changed.

It is the first day of what is meant to be a blissful, much-needed, two-week break from law school after a recent round of intense exams. But what starts out as a slightly self-indulgent, incredibly geeky trip to WHSmith to stock up on brand-new stationery (I never claimed I was cool!) ends in tragedy. Still riding high from my triumphant purchase of what I deem to be the ultimate highlighter pen set, I walk through the automatic doors at the front of the shop and, as I do, my eyes flick down to my phone. The screen flashes up with ten missed calls from my brother and eight from my mum.

This is not normal.

My first thought is that there must be something wrong with my phone. I've rarely, if ever, been this in demand in my entire life (save for maybe that time when all my university housemates concurrently forgot, lost or had otherwise misplaced their own house keys) and certainly not on a very ordinary Monday morning and with multiple members of my family simultaneously. I call my brother as I make my way back to my car. He doesn't answer, so I try again. This time he answers in an uncharacteristically quiet voice, with only four short words that turn me upside down, rip me inside out and break me apart on the spot.

'Dad's died, come home.'

Every sound is loud. Too loud, bouncing uncomfortably off my eardrums.

The light, that only a few moments before I had been admiring, is now too bright; it burns the back of my eyes.

I'm confused. He can't have said 'Dad'; I must have misheard. He's not dead, he's alive. I only saw him yesterday when he came to visit me. We had Sunday lunch together; he gave me a hug and told me he loved me (which happens to be the first time in my life I can ever recall either of these things happening). He's not unwell, he's young; he's only 56.

No, I think to myself, he must have said 'Grandad'. Yes, that was it, Grandad must have died. That's the only thing that makes logical sense as my maternal grandfather has been in and out of hospital for a while now. But although my brother is no longer on the phone, his voice is still ringing clearly in my ears – 'Dad', he had definitely said 'Dad'.

Dad has died.

All sounds have stopped now, the air is still.

I'm walking, my feet are moving, but I don't recall making the decision to ask them to move. I don't cry, but I feel like I'm wading through thick, sticky mud.

'Jo, are you OK?' A familiar voice snaps me back to reality.

I have walked pretty much smack bang into my then housemate.

'Err... no, I'm not,' I stammer. Unsure of what to say next, I blurt out, 'My dad's just died, and I think... I need to go home to Mum.'

'Oh... errr... right. Yes... OK.' I hear her stumble over her words. I see my own fear mirrored on her face, I see my shock reflected as her eyes widen and her face greys.

And just like that, my life is forever changed. My world will always be split into two distinct parts. Sliced cleanly in half. I am eternally divided into before this day and what comes after it. Pre- to post-. Present tense to past tense. Alive to dead.

It will be weeks yet before we find out what Dad died of. Tragically, it was a burst stomach ulcer that would have been very much treatable had it been caught earlier. But it had lain undetected like an undiscovered bomb ticking silently away deep within him. Its slight discomfort was chalked up to a stressful job and something that would abate on his pending early retirement later that year, only for the bomb to explode and for him to be torn away from us with alarming speed.

♥ JOS' TOOLKIT: WHAT TO DO WHEN A FRIEND IS MOURNING

▸ *Don't call.* When someone dies you suddenly find yourself spending an exhausting amount of time on the phone, talking to close relatives, telling acquaintances, sorting the inordinately long list of death admin that needs to be undertaken. Don't add to this list.

▸ *Write them a card or a note.* Don't text – like phone calls, the number of texts received at times like these is numerous and overwhelming. And how do you even begin to respond anyway? 'Thanks' feels forced and weird. Don't worry if you don't know what to say and your words will probably feel clunky. Write them anyway. Say you don't know what to say. Something is better than nothing. Tell them you love them. Tell them you care about them. Tell them you will continue to be there in the years to come. And then follow through and actually continue to be there in the years to come. The hardest times are often when the initial hubbub has died down, the visitors and messages have stopped coming, and your mourning is supposed to be over, perhaps before it has even begun. Some friends of mine for many years after my dad died sent flowers to my work on the anniversary of his death. They will never know how much this tiny but enormously kind gesture meant to me.

▸ *Do not expect a response.* Tell them you neither want nor expect a response – now is not the time for them to feel any extra burden of politeness.

- ▶ *Don't buy them flowers.* If you feel compelled to get them something, buy them a vase (grieving people often find themselves with an excess of flowers and a deficit of things to put them in).

- ▶ *Offer to tell mutual friends or family* who may not have heard.

- ▶ *Offer to mend things around the house* – a disproportionate number of things seem to break, stop working or need fixing when there is a death in the household.

Late that night, after I have returned to the family home and the chaotic and frenzied energy of the day has stilled slightly, I turn the events of the day over and over in my mind. The phone call, the journey back, the disbelief turning into realisation and splintering pain. The extra layer of heartbreak I feel when I see so clearly in my mum's eyes my grief. I can't stand it, it's too much to bear.

It's as if a switch has been flicked inside me and, in an instant, aged 23, I become my mum's mother. I make a decision that night to pack away my grief in a suitcase in my mind, labelled neatly 'for later'. I feel an all-consuming duty to my dad to be strong for her, to look after her, to protect her from any extra hurt. It's as if his voice fills my head telling me this is what I should do. I feel grateful that I have a purpose, that I have his guidance. Because, for now, I have a focus. I must be there for my mum. I am fine, I am calm, I am doing what Dad would want. I will hold her together, I will hold us both together.

THERAPY IS EXCRUCIATING

A few weeks go by and I need to return to law school for one final term, and I throw myself back into my studies, my friends, going out, getting drunk, boys and appearing 'normal'.

I haven't even begun to start the grieving process; I am firmly stuck on the first of Elisabeth Kübler-Ross's five stages of grief. And there I will stubbornly stay, with denial as my close friend, comfort and most effective numbing agent, for at least the next decade or so.

My law school has told me I must have at least six counselling sessions in order to fulfil their duty of care. I can't see the point myself and I don't want to go. I don't need this. I have friends, plenty of them. Fickle, fun ones who help me forget, but also real, true ones who offer wide shoulders for crying and open ears for listening should I need them. If I wanted or needed to talk to anyone, I have my friends.

I don't talk to them of course, but that's not the point. I could, right?

JO'S TOOLKIT: HOW TALKING TO A GOOD THERAPIST IS DIFFERENT TO TALKING TO A FRIEND

I wish I could go back and tell myself that therapy is not a replacement for friendship nor is it an indication of any failure to make good friends. In fact, having now experienced the wonderful way great therapy actually works, I know we cannot expect our friends, however empathetic they may be, however amazing they are at listening, to consistently and persistently put their own needs to one side in order to service ours.

I wish I had known:

▶ Conversation is just the surface level of therapy: good therapy delves far deeper than chatting to a friend can do.

▶ A great therapist will challenge your thinking so you can try new ways of improving your life. They are on your team, but they won't *always* agree with you.

▶ Friends can be great at listening and giving advice BUT only a therapist has the skills and years of training to help improve your mental health without risking any damage to your personal relationships.

▶ A skilled therapist will be objective and unbiased as they have no emotional stake in your relationship the way friends do, however lovely they might be.

▶ Therapists will keep your secrets, friends may do but then again they may not!

▶ You don't need to feel guilty or a burden for taking up too much of your therapist's time or feel you need to give them the same amount of support in return.

▶ A therapist has spent years training to refrain from judgement. If you share something intense, even a sensitive friend might react in a way that you don't want them to or that hurts either of your feelings.

▶ However open we are with our friends we often present only a version of ourselves to them, meaning we tiptoe around or avoid altogether certain topics that we are not prepared to show our friends but can happily let our therapists see.

▶ Talking to a friend may be free in terms of money spent, but there often is a price to pay. Free therapy from a friend could end up costing you that friendship and more.

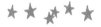

The counselling all starts with me filling out a questionnaire, with questions such as:

▶ Have your sleeping patterns changed considerably since the death of your loved one?

▶ Has your weight changed considerably since the death of your loved one?

▶ Have you experienced great or regular confusion since the death of your loved one?

▶ Have you been unable to stop crying since the death of your loved one?

▶ Have you been unable to concentrate since the death of your loved one?

All of these get a neat tick in the 'no' box, not because I have acknowledged my thoughts and feelings about my dad's death or am working through them in healthy ways, as this counsellor suggests, but because I haven't even begun to process any of it.

We sit for long, painful stretches in complete toe-curling silence.

I 'um' and 'ah' a lot. I can't get comfortable and shift around in my seat.

I ask her what we are supposed to talk about. She frowns and wonders aloud why I need her permission or guidance to do or say anything. I flinch at her words and feel suitably scolded. Eventually, when she is met with more silence, her answer, rather unhelpfully for me, is 'Whatever you want to talk about.'

But I don't want.

So we go back to silence.

It is excruciatingly uncomfortable. Her just looking at me makes me feel exposed.

And this is how most of our sessions play out, with barely a single word said by either of us. The heavy weight of expectation on me to say something, to say anything, drags me down and paralyses me. I feel like I am under the sharp glare of a spotlight, a specimen in a Petri dish being examined.

She says I can talk about anything, but I know this isn't really true. It's the elephant in the room, the spectre of which hangs unspoken in the air between us. She knows why I am actually here, I know why I am here and what, or more specifically who, I'm supposed to be talking about and I can't. I deeply resent any attempt to unlock my war-torn inner world.

I am trapped.

But yet we stagger on, cringing through session after session, because we both know we have to. Our painful slots are endured, the rules have told us so, and I guess, looking back, it was probably almost as agonising for her as it was for me.

Our largely wordless sessions eventually come to an end, and life for me carries on much as it did before. And all the while, my grief is like a bruise on the secret centre of my being that I carry with me everywhere I go, excruciatingly tender to the touch but locked in too deep for anyone else to see.

Many years would pass before this bruise would begin to be exposed to the light and start to heal, its vivid colours fading from purple, to blue, to pink, but never leaving me entirely. But back then I did not want to be made to mourn what I had lost. I resisted it not only in the counsellor's office, but in all corners of my life and with every fibre of my being.

JO'S TOOLKIT: THINGS NO ONE TELLS YOU WHEN YOU LOSE A LOVED ONE

1   It can be surprisingly tough when people ask you simple questions about your family like 'Where do they live?'/'What do they do?' and you have to carefully use past-tense verbs for those who are no longer with you, hoping the other person won't notice or delve further.

2   You might find you have a strong reaction when your friends casually complain about their family. What you would do for one more annoying phone call or cringey joke in a cheesy text message.

3   Father's Day or Mothering Sunday are super hard as you're bombarded with 'perfect gift ideas', email marketing campaigns popping uninvited into your inbox and social media feeds filled for 24 hours with gushing posts that are all incredibly painful reminders that you'll never get another chance just to tell them that you love them.

4   Of course, all the major life milestones are hard to navigate too – getting your dream job, meeting the love of your life, getting married, having kids are all tinged with sadness as you long to share it with them.

5   It's hard when you think to yourself, 'I haven't spoken to that person in a while, I had better call them,' and then you remember you can't.

6   It's tough when you catch a glimpse of someone in the street who carries themselves in the same way, looks similar or reminds you of them in some way and your grief smacks you in the chest.

7   It's tough when you hear songs from their funeral or wake come on the radio. The one that regularly gets me is 'Johnny B. Goode' by Chuck Berry, which seems to be played on the dance floor at pretty much every single wedding I've attended since my dad died.

The remainder of my twenties is smoke and mirrors. Nothing is as it seems. I am not as I seem.

I walk a fine line every day, making it appear as if I have it all together when all the while internally I am breaking apart. By day, my Louboutins clip down the corridors of a fancy City law firm in London and by night, I am raising glasses in the plushest of cocktail bars and pilgrimaging to the most exclusive of members' clubs. The outside world sees me as a plugged in, successful, healthy person. But it's not the truth, it's all a distraction, a veneer. The façade of having it all is flimsy yet surprisingly effective at deflecting scrutiny, while behind my fortress of control the self-destruct button has been pushed.

I wake each morning with feelings of impending doom, only to push those feelings down in any way I can find. I work, too much. I drink, too much. I go out, too much. I diet, too much. I spend, too much. I exercise, too much. It all swirls around me like the heady dance of a drunken merry-go-round. I have no balance, no counterweight, no anchor. I dive deep into the pool of distraction so I don't have to confront my feelings. But they follow me wherever I go like a sticky shadow, in the dimly lit nightclub bathroom, at my desk at work, lurking on the edges of every effort to rub myself clean of them.

The pervasive need to control each tick of the clock seeps into everything I do. Every ounce of energy is devoted to it. All around me I see versions of myself that are better, prettier, smarter, something more. I see my flaws everywhere; snatched reflections of a distorted fun-house mirror version of myself. My life has turned into a game of hiding who I really am under a cloak of perfectionism. I have become my accomplishments; I am my career, my salary, my weight, my wardrobe; I am what I do; I am what I have; I am what I achieve; and I am what other people think of me.

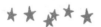

When eventually, more than a decade later, I tell my therapist that it feels as though the grief is so locked up inside it may never come out, she explains she can help and that we are going to do the 'empty chair' technique. She tells me to focus on the empty chair in the corner of her room and picture my father sitting there across from me.

The years since I last saw his face make this incredibly hard as the memories that once seemed so permanent have blurred, become fuzzy and just outside of my grasp. I scrunch up my face and search around in my memory trying to conjure up the image of him before me. How is this so hard? Have I forgotten him completely? What a betrayal that would be.

And just as my therapist is gently asking me to think of some details about him – what he might be wearing, how he would be sitting, etc. – I see his hands. Just like that, there they are. Large and comforting, knuckles weathered and coarse. I didn't know that I knew their detail in the way that I do. They are something so intimate. Something so known.

And with this, something deep, deep inside of me is finally unleashed. It's as though the very essence of him roars around me. It's not just the hands now – there he is exactly as he's always been, quietly sitting, watching me as my grief bubbles up and pours uncontrollably out of me. The tears have finally arrived.

Therapy thoughts

'Sometimes, you need an objective ear. Friends tend to automatically take your side or bring their own agenda to a conversation. In therapy, you have someone who doesn't know you intimately and can help you gain clarity.'

Natasha Devon MBE, mental health and body image campaigner and writer

Chapter Three
THERAPY IS
Overwhelming

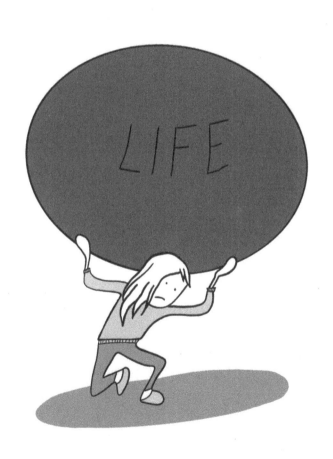

My pregnancy was unexpected, complicated and largely joyless. We hadn't been trying for a baby, but after too many years of being on contraception I'd decided my physical and mental health might benefit from a break. However, my usual careful calculations were overlooked during a hedonistic week in Ibiza and we headed home with more than just sore heads and cases of 'Ibiza flu' – a secret little pip had taken hold inside of me.

I don't think I ever overcame the shock of my pregnancy. I didn't find out I was pregnant until I was nearly 10 weeks... Bella then burst, dramatically and rather traumatically, into our lives almost three weeks early, leaving me just over 20 weeks, rather than the usual 40, for processing what the hell was happening. It turns out this was not enough time.

LOSING CONTROL

I've not slept properly since the day Bella was born. Roughly 300 sleepless nights later and it feels like the cracks in my brain have become deep cavernous sinkholes swallowing up old parts of myself permanently.

She cries more than she doesn't.

I cry too.

Often.

But mostly I am numb. I feel like a ghost. I don't feel like I am really here, as though I have faded away. For the past few weeks I have really begun to feel like I might be losing my mind; my thoughts are persistently negative and often not rooted in reality.

I feel as if I'm wearing many heavy coats that don't belong to me – coats of domesticity, unrelenting responsibility and martyrdom weighing me down, keeping me hidden, engulfing me with their enormous bulk. I have to get motherhood right, tick all the boxes, do all the classes, batch cook all the food, research all the stages, do it all, and above all be selflessly perfect even if that means I cease to exist in the process.

Selfless.

Self.

Less.

To be without oneself.

I am definitely without my self.

I have lost myself entirely. I don't know who I am anymore.

During the week I fixate on the time my husband, Chris, is due home: half past six. I tell myself I have to hold it together until then.

With all my might.

If the minute hand ticks past this time, the anxiety rises inside me like a rocket. My heart beats faster; I struggle to breathe. Stuck in traffic or a puncture on his bike, a meeting that overruns, a chat on the way out of the office with a colleague... anything that delays him by mere minutes means he arrives home to a sobbing, shaking wreck.

As a result, I pin all my focus for any kind of reprieve on the weekends, where I believe I will magically gain some precious time and feel a little bit normal again. But the reality never lives up to the expectation, there is no 'normal' to be regained, and the cycle of unrelenting duties continues.

This is just par for the motherhood course. Everyone feels like this, they can just cope with it a bit better, I reason to myself.

But my world exists in great grey layers of thick, cold fog.

I've finally lost control, the momentum of the spinning merry-go-round has become too much. I can no longer hold on.

I am flailing.

I am flung.

And if I'm honest, I've not felt in control for the longest time.

JO'S TOOLKIT: HOW TO HELP NEW MUMS

▶ *Never turn up expectedly.* It's highly likely you'll be interrupting something: the nappy change of all nappy changes (no more needs to be said on that one), bath time (an often overlooked detail, but it is literally impossible to leave a baby in the bath while you run and answer the door), a much-needed moment of peace or, heaven forbid, a naptime or bedtime (never ever put yourself at risk of this one – the repercussions of a sleeping baby interrupted too early is never a fun thing to have to deal with).

▶ *Never knock on the door or ring the bell.* Always text or call when you're outside. If you wake a sleeping baby, on your head be it (see above)!

▶ *Preferably you should make food, any food.* Take it over and leave it on the doorstep. Don't offer to share it with them and do not ask to come in. And I repeat – do NOT knock on the door or ring the bell!

▶ *If you are invited in, make yourself useful.* Even if they protest, never let the new parent play host. Wash up; feed the dog, cat, budgie; empty the dishwasher; entertain the older kids; wipe the table; sort the washing. Look around – see what needs to be done.

▶ *Never overstay your welcome.* If in doubt, leave well before you think you should.

- *Watch the baby* – offer to take the buggy to the park, down the street, round the block. Or simply sit with the baby while Mum has a nap upstairs, a shower, even a wee!

- *Get them an audiobook* or recommendations, podcast suggestions or a playlist. Crucially these can all be enjoyed hands-free as a new mum's hands are never free.

WHAT NOT TO SAY TO A NEW MUM…

Is he/she a 'good' baby? Sleeping through the night yet?

I'm coming over right now.

Enjoy every moment; you'll miss it when they are grown.

TRY THIS INSTEAD…

How are you feeling? What do you need right now?

I'm going food shopping later, anything you need? I'll drop over some food. I'll leave it on the doorstep. No need to come out.

It can be really hard. I'm here and I'm listening if you need to offload.

From the Other Chair
PERINATAL ILLNESS

As Dr Emma Hepburn, clinical psychologist (aka @thepsychologymum on Instagram), explains, a 'perinatal' mental health difficulty is one that someone might experience any time from becoming pregnant up to a year after they give birth. This may be a new mental health concern or something they've experienced in the past.

Having a baby is a big life event. It's natural to experience a range of emotions during pregnancy and after giving birth. Having the 'baby blues' after giving birth is very common. Symptoms can include feeling emotional and irrational, bursting into tears for no apparent reason, feeling irritable or touchy, feeling depressed or anxious. Baby blues tend to start in the week after birth and usually only last a few days. These feelings are very normal and are not an indication of a perinatal mental health illness. However, if these feelings are very severe or last more than two weeks it could be a sign someone might be experiencing postnatal depression or another perinatal mental health difficulty.

Postnatal depression
Postnatal depression can start at any time in the first year after giving birth and might develop very gradually. Therefore, many women do not always realise that they are experiencing it. Your midwife or health visitor will normally screen for depression using a measure such as the Edinburgh Postnatal Depression Scale. It can range from mild to very severe. Symptoms will vary from person to person, but you might experience feeling:

- hostile or indifferent towards your baby or partner

- hopeless

- isolated or lost

- a lack of self-esteem or confidence

- numbness or emptiness

- no pleasure or joy in things you used to enjoy

- sad, down, upset or tearful

- guilt, shame or worthlessness

- mood swings, irritability, aggression or anger

- agitation or restlessness

- suicidal

Other perinatal mental health concerns

Postnatal depression is not the only perinatal mental health concern, but it is probably the best known. There are other mental health difficulties that many people experience during pregnancy or in the first year after birth, and it is not uncommon to experience more than one simultaneously. Some of these are:

- antenatal (while pregnant) depression or anxiety

- perinatal anxiety

- perinatal OCD

- postpartum psychosis

▶ postpartum PTSD and birth trauma

▶ some women also experience eating problems during and after pregnancy

---

I'm sitting in my bedroom on a Saturday afternoon. Bella is finally sleeping in her cot after what feels like yet another soul-destroying battle of wills when Chris declares he is going for a run. This is enough for me to feel as though I am unravelling. Quietly though, so as to not wake the baby of course, but I can feel the sobs pulsing in my chest, the tightening and heaving. Inside I'm screaming, spiralling deep into an inky destructive rage.

A run.

Sounds simple enough on the surface, right? It should be fine – I know that now of course, now that I'm not unwell, now I'm not struggling to breathe under all the heavy coats I'm wearing. But at the time it isn't fine, in fact it is the very last thing from being fine.

He is escaping, he is leaving the house. He isn't asking either, he is telling me. How dare he leave me here alone, and on a weekend too. Why has he not got the memo that this is the only time I have to rest? Can he not see that I am the one who needs to escape, needs a break, needs to be free?

Despite living under the same roof, our worlds at this moment in time couldn't feel further apart. The thought of me saying, 'I'm going out of the house alone' is alien to me, almost otherworldly. I know on one level that I too could say I am going for a run, but in the same breath I know that I can't. I can't leave. I don't even shower these days, most days my teeth don't get cleaned as it all feels too much effort, so it is unfathomable to me how I'd find the energy or impetus to be able to tackle the seemingly herculean task of a run. I feel duty-bound to look after the tiny human we have made.

Yet I feel trapped. I am drowning. I am a husk.

'I need a break. I need everything to stop,' I hiss under my breath, hoping the baby stays sleeping.

'What kind of break?' I hear him ask, his voice cracking with pain.

It takes me a moment, but I eventually realise he thinks I mean a divorce.

I don't mean a divorce. Well I don't think I mean a divorce. I rummage through my mind and every wounded pore of my body, desperately searching for a clearer understanding of this idea that even I don't fully grasp myself.

'I don't know,' I finally admit.

And I don't know. I don't know what 'a break' means. It's not a holiday. It's not a spa day. It's this massive, impossible desire to put the whole world on pause so I can rest. The agony of emotional paralysis, the desperation for an unknown something without the slightest idea of what that might be, and the ever-present need for everything to stop. Beyond stop, to be lost, be forgotten entirely.

To disappear.

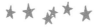

Years later, I have revisited this moment and how I unravelled about the run many times over in and out of the therapy room, and I have been able to diffuse the emotional heat from it almost entirely. I'll touch later in this book on how, with the help of a brilliant therapist, I was able to heal this wound, but, needless to say, at the time, the energy of this moment is still burning and ripping through my veins as I hear the slam of the door below as my husband makes his bid for freedom.

I remain seated on my bed. I know I need to stand up and pretend everything is OK, pretend that I am OK, because the tiny heartbeat and gentle breath coming from the cot nearby needs me to. But I can't, something inside has given up. I stay sitting, I am calcified, my bones fused like lead to the bed.

It's a cold bright day and I can hear the hum of London life on the street outside; children playing somewhere nearby, cars passing, the dull drone of machinery of some sort off in the distance.

The painkillers that I have been robotically and unconsciously squirrelling away for 'when I need them' are piled on my hand.

I look at the array I've collected, more than 20 I guess at a glance, maybe 30.

'That should be enough,' I reason.

Enough.

'Enough for what?' I think.

Enough to take this pain away, enough to allow my family to be better off without me, enough to disappear.

I long to disappear.

I stare at their different shapes and sizes. The chalky white coating of many, the smoother surfaces of others, their grooves, their edges, the tiny words on some, the ruby-red shiny gleaming bubbles of others. I think to myself they look like tiny, potent, toxic jewels. I can still to this day feel the weight of those pills in my hand, remember the chalky residue they left in their wake.

I don't know what breaks the spell, maybe it's a noise outside, maybe it's Chris returning from his run, maybe Bella shifts in her cot, reconnecting that maternal rope. Maybe it's the thought that doing nothing is somehow easier than doing something.

But the bubble bursts; I scrape the pills into the drawer and vow to get help.

From the Other Chair
CRISIS SUPPORT

As Dr Rebecca Moore, co-founder of Make Birth Better, explains, suicidal thoughts are surprisingly common, particularly if you are a new mum. Suicide is one of the leading causes of death among women occurring within a year after the end of pregnancy.

If you're feeling like you want to die, harm or hurt yourself, the first thing to say is please know you're not alone. The most important thing to do if you feel like this is to talk about it. The better able we are to talk about these feelings, the less likely we are to act on them.

It might feel really hard, but try to let family or friends know what's going on for you. They may be able to offer support and help keep you safe. There's no right or wrong way to talk about suicidal feelings – starting the conversation is what's important.

If you find it difficult to talk to someone you know, you could:

▶ Phone a helpline like the Samaritans on 116 123 (more are listed on page 260).

▶ Talk to a health professional, your GP, midwife or health visitor.

▶ Text SHOUT (85258) for free text message support 24/7.

▶ Call 111 (the NHS non-emergency line) – they will help you find the support and help you need. Note, sometimes it is possible to speak to a qualified mental health nurse through this line.

▶ Call 999 or go to your local A&E.

▶ Contact your mental health crisis team, if you have one.

For more crisis resources, please see page 260.

A LIFELINE

It's raining as I wheel the buggy to yet another baby class. Before I know what I have done, I have diverted the wheels into the open doors of the doctors' waiting room and am now sat waiting for my name to be called, the rain cover slowly dripping on to my already soaked jeans. And, of course, the baby is crying. All eyes are staring at me. Judgement sears into my bones.

'I get being a mum is hard,' I say to the friendly face staring expectantly at me, 'but should it be this hard?' I ask, fighting back the tears, determined not to completely lose it in front of yet another GP, desperately trying to keep my voice steady against the hard, immovable lump that's suddenly appeared in it. A knowing look darts across her face for a second and then is gone.

'I don't think it should be, no,' she says, as she tots up the scores to a series of questions that I now know to be the Edinburgh Scale to diagnose postnatal depression. 'I think we need to talk about medication and therapy.'

There it is again. The power couple of shame, the dynamic duo of disgrace – medication and therapy.

But this time it's different. This time I don't fight them.

I have run out of energy, I am at rock bottom, drowning, and I know I need all the lifelines I can get. Yet while I accept them in, oh how I feel like I have failed as a human and as a mother.

Five years on and a slightly different picture has thankfully emerged, with the Internet offering a crucial platform to speak up about these issues and extend solidarity to mums in their darkest moments. However, the sea of frank stories about 'what nobody tells you about parenthood' has potentially now tipped us too far the other way. One friend recently told me that the efforts now being made not to sugar-coat the difficulties of modern parenting online are in fact deterring many, including herself, from having children. Not to trivialise what I and others who have developed maternal mental health issues have experienced, but I think the reality of what most mothers will go through in the first years of motherhood is often somewhere in between the horror stories and the perfectly curated social media feeds. Something along the lines of 'It's not always going to be easy, but it's going to be all right.' But boy, it was not easy.

JO'S TOOLKIT: TALKING TO A DOCTOR ABOUT YOUR MENTAL HEALTH

Talking to a doctor about mental health can be really tough. I have often found myself downplaying my symptoms when I am faced with a professional. Instead of remembering how awful I felt the days and weeks before, I find that self-doubt and embarrassment creep in and it's easier to mumble vaguely about how I haven't been feeling great recently. And when they probe a bit further or give me a quizzical look – because, let's be honest, today I have somehow managed to assemble myself into someone who looks like a functioning member of society – I start to question myself even more. I feel a pressure to say something like, 'I suppose it's normal, I suppose everyone feels sad sometimes. I'm just a bit stressed right now. Yes, I'm OK really, I'm sure it will pass.' And then I leave, wondering what the hell just happened. Why do I now feel so instantly crushed and like I'm drowning again? Why did I say I was OK when I'm really not? Why wasn't I strong enough to articulate my feelings? Why did I crumble so quickly? I was there, I had hold of the life ring, why the hell did I let it go?

If you've found yourself with similar feelings, the next time you're feeling sad, alone, anxious, scared, not yourself, like you can't go on, get out your phone and write down what you're feeling right in that moment. Even if it's just one word. Take this to your next appointment, either to remind you or literally to hand to the doctor if that's easier. Your main job is to get across to them that what you're experiencing isn't normal for you. And remember you are ultimately the best judge of knowing what is normal *for you*, and what is not.

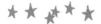

I feel so ashamed collecting my prescription for my antidepressants and, despite no one in the queue behind me being able to read the tiny words printed on the slip of green paper that I have just thrust over the counter, their restless disapproving energy bores into my back as if they can.

The young pharmacist's eyes scan me up and down in what I take to be silent damnation. I feel the double whammy of failure and shame flush through my body.

Later that day I take the tiny white tablets and within only a few days I start to feel lighter. Smiles that had been missing for so long start appearing. My patience grows stronger, the fog starts to lift, the colour slowly starts to return.

Within weeks, I feel almost like my old self again.

Almost, but not quite.

From the Other Chair
ANTIDEPRESSANTS

As Dr Sarah Vohra, consultant psychiatrist (aka @themindmedic on Instagram), explains, antidepressants are a type of medicine used to treat clinical depression. There are several different types of antidepressants. Selective serotonin reuptake inhibitors (SSRIs) are the most widely prescribed and are usually preferred over other antidepressants as they cause fewer side effects. Antidepressants work by making certain chemicals in our brains called neurotransmitters (involved in regulating our mood) more available. They can help lift mood, increase energy and concentration levels, and improve appetite and sleep, which can help you cope better with day-to-day life – something that previously may have been too challenging or difficult. However, while antidepressants can help treat the symptoms of depression, they do not always address the cause and therefore are usually used in combination with other treatments such as therapy.

JO'S TOOLKIT: TEN THINGS NO ONE TELLS YOU ABOUT TAKING ANTIDEPRESSANTS

▶ Antidepressants work differently for different people. Don't think that what works for others will necessarily work for you.

▶ Sometimes it requires a lot of trial and error to find the right fit. Don't give up.

▶ Taking medication for a mental illness is just like doing so for any physical illness. You wouldn't question taking medication to heal an issue with, say, your liver – there should be no difference with a different organ, your brain.

▶ They aren't magic pills that make you happy all the time.

▶ The first few days or weeks on antidepressants might be a little rocky.

▶ You don't necessarily need to be on them forever.

▶ If you do need to be on them for a long time, there's nothing wrong with that.

▶ But remember that feeling better doesn't necessarily mean you should stop taking them. NEVER think you can do this alone, always speak to your doctor first. Trust me, stopping your medication without support is no fun whatsoever. Keep taking your meds!

▶ They're not meant to turn you into a zombie.

▶ Taking antidepressants does not make you weak. You are doing what you need to suffer less, so you can live more. This makes you a goddamn hero.

THERAPY IS SELF-INDULGENT

In our short course of CBT sessions my new therapist, Cara, tells me she wants to focus on positive goals and breaking my negative thought patterns.

'That sounds OK to me,' I think to myself, but I can't shake the feeling that I shouldn't be here. I've been taking my medication for over two months now and I feel OK. I feel like I'm wasting not only my own time, but valuable NHS resources, and despite being suicidal mere weeks ago, I can't stop feeling I'm not poorly enough and this is too egotistical. There are people out there who have things so much worse, who I am to complain? I feel like a middle-class cliché, unable to cope with my objectively perfectly lovely life and now self-indulgently blathering away about myself on a weekly basis.

This imposter feeling hasn't been helped by a couple of recent experiences.

The first is a comment made by a nurse at a routine appointment. Upon hearing I am on antidepressants for postnatal depression, she tells me that I shouldn't be, my child is too old for me to have postnatal depression. I know she is wrong, I know she is mixing it up with the baby blues. But even though I know she's made a mistake, she is a nurse, she is the professional and maybe it is me who is wrong. After all, my mind hasn't felt like my own recently. She has me rattled and I am now questioning myself.

The second is a passing, almost imperceptible aside, muttered by a friend when I mention I'm starting therapy. 'What a luxury', she whistles on an outbreath. Whether she meant me to hear or not, her three little words pack their toxic shameful punch all the same.

Cara asks me to keep notes of my thoughts and behaviours on a daily basis and bring them in to therapy for review. This is the first nail in the coffin for me. I desperately want to please her; I want to get this right, I want to be a good client. My need to shape-shift and people-please rallies against my bone-deep exhaustion. Does she not know how all-consuming this time of my life is? Homework feels just too tedious. Too cumbersome. Too irrelevant to a mother yearning for a moment's peace. This feels far too much like hard work, and frankly, who feels like doing homework when you are sleep-deprived?

So I fudge it. I spin tales only loosely related to the life I'm leading. I tell her I am fine, I bring her my funniest stories, my shiniest parts. I want her to laugh at my anecdotes, see that I'm actually completely fine. It's not all totally false; the medication is helping convince me of this too, much of the time. I long for her to tell me how well I am doing. How it was all a big misunderstanding and actually I can go freely back into the world with a shiny gold star feeling great about myself again.

Except, she sees through me. Of course she does, and she doesn't just see, she holds a mirror up to my behaviour.

'Jo, you say you're fine, but you're not. I think you need to spend some time reflecting on whether our time together is beneficial to you.' She starts gently, but now there is a sterner edge creeping in: 'I don't think you've been truthful to me about what's going on in your life, and ultimately I think this is interfering with your progress and wasting both of our time.'

I am offended. I do not like it one little bit.

I feel myself suddenly getting unexplainable hot prickles of what feel like they might be tears in my eyes. I will them away. 'Who died and made you so goddamn perfect?' I yell, inside my head of course. Outwardly I mutter that I don't know what she means, even though I know exactly what she means. I flush with embarrassment, shuffle my feet and don't know what else to say. I know in that moment that I will never come back to this cosy little room and see this warm and intuitive woman. And just like that another therapist bites the proverbial dust and I'm on my own again.

But I'm fine, totally fine, I tell myself silently on a loop.

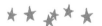

The idea of spending dozens of weeks (and in many cases thousands of pounds) discussing your neuroses can feel and look like a self-indulgent luxury. It can seem selfish to spend so much time looking at your navel through a microscope when there are people in the world with far more pressing problems.

And when you take the long waiting lists and high price point into account, therapy feels even more of a luxury. But it shouldn't be. There is no hierarchy of woe, in which some conditions of life are inherently more misery-making than others. Life is relative – what might be a serious problem for you may be easy for me to cope with, or vice versa.

Pursuing therapy is a sign of strength, not weakness. We all need help from time to time; if I have a bad tooth, I go to the dentist; if my car breaks down, I go to the mechanic. We get professional support for all kinds of problems, and mental health is no different.

THERAPY IS NECESSARY

There is something that keeps pulling me back to therapy despite many less-than-perfect experiences in the therapy room. It's as if there is an invisible rope that is winding me back in time and again, as I repeatedly ignore it and slam myself full force into rock bottom.

It is as if therapy keeps showing up, patiently holding out its hand for me to grab it and take hold. After all other options have been exhausted, it is still there diligently waiting for me to heal my wounds.

It's at this point in the book I wish there was a way to insert the literary equivalent of a fanfare, or a klaxon, or even a line of chorus girls dancing across the page to signify to you, the reader, of an important upcoming plot point.

Around this time and quite by accident, I discover I am entitled to six sessions with a therapist under a long-forgotten-about health insurance policy. Sod it, I think, what have I got to lose? I do a little research this time, read a few bios (for more on how to find a therapist and my tips on the process, skip ahead to Chapter Ten), make a few phone calls and, before I know it, I have an appointment to see someone the following week.

And, just like that, into my life walks Elinor, aka 'The One' [chorus girls exit stage left].

Her office is simple but comfortable, in one of those 'posh sheds' at the end of the garden. It backs on to a primary school playing field, meaning our conversations are often accompanied by the riotous and strangely comforting sound of children playing nearby. I always sit directly opposite her facing a long, pleasant garden in the middle of a comfortable, dark grey, L-shaped sofa, where I manage to half bury myself in the bright colourful cushions with bold leafy patterns. And crucially, unlike previous therapists, both she and her office smell pretty good. This is definitely an unexpected bonus.

Beneath my feet is a rug with various grey, white and blue geometric shapes on it. I spend a lot of time over the years looking at this rug, as well as out of the door behind Elinor's head watching the slow change of the seasons as the weeks tick by. I take these things in, not in awkward fixation as I have done in previous therapists' offices or as a way to avoid eye contact, but merely in moments of pause, contemplation or just observing the space around me as we talk.

As I cast my mind back to Elinor's homely garden office, I am overcome with an intense wave of nostalgia for this private, protected space. And I realise now, as I sit and type these words, that not only did she purposefully and nurturingly spin a cocoon of safety, warmth and trust into this physical space, but she did it around me emotionally too.

REASONS ELINOR IS 'THE ONE'

1   *I feel safe*. She offers a consistent, confidential, caring space for me to explore my innermost feelings.

2   *I don't bullshit her*. I will hold my hands up here, it's true, I do want her to like me, but I find that this doesn't get in the way of being able to talk to her truthfully. I don't just bring my shiniest parts for her approval, instead I am able to say what is going on for me, even when those thoughts and feelings don't make me look so great.

3 *She doesn't bullshit me.* I remember her telling me in our very first session, quite matter of factly, that it is perfectly OK if I decide we aren't the right fit for each other. She also warns me there will be times when it will be hard and there are also likely to be times I won't like her very much. She says it will be uncomfortable to hear myself say out loud things I've never voiced before, not even to my closest friends. She explains this is not only OK, it is completely normal.

4 *I feel heard and understood.* Opening the rawest, ugliest parts of myself to someone new is pretty terrifying. But instead of judgement or criticism, I feel empathy and validation. She truly listens to me and it is empowering.

5 *It's a two-way street.* She walks alongside me and it feels as though she is accompanying me rather than observing me. She works collaboratively with me, encouraging me to find my own answers, but never leaving me to wander alone.

6 *It's not a chore.* I find even when it starts getting tough and we tap into the more difficult experiences or emotions, it never feels like a chore. In fact, I start to look forward to my sessions and the sense of relief they bring.

It is now, in the safety of Elinor's garden cocoon, that the talking really begins. Word by word, topic by topic, I tentatively and slowly unwrap the layers of myself, baring to her my worries, my fears, my pain.

Elinor and I talk about my family, we talk about my dad's death, we talk about my childhood, we talk about my desire to break the cycle of generational trauma we all pass on to our kids. We speak about my little girl, we talk about the postnatal depression, we talk about how I still feel I can't cope; I tell her about how I can't look at photographs of Bella as a baby without my heart feeling like it has been ripped from my chest with regret, guilt and self-loathing. We talk through my ideas of how I think motherhood should look and how I almost destroyed myself trying to achieve it. We talk about issues I'm having in some of my friendships, how I feel as if I am a fundamentally deeply unlikable human and how I will turn myself inside out trying to be liked and receive external validation. We talk about how acutely uncomfortable I am with saying no. We talk about how lost I feel, and at a snail's pace, side by side, we begin to piece the misunderstood, misplaced, neglected and unloved parts of myself back together.

It's as if together we are archaeologists of my past, patiently and diligently excavating my mind, sifting through layers of painful memories and trauma, exposing long-buried secrets and links. Me with the hammer blindly bashing through layers of emotional dirt, Elinor with her brush, carefully and gently dusting off each emotional artefact and examining it for meaning and connection to my present self.

I repeat myself often. Sometimes within a session, but, more often than not, similar topics and themes are brought up again and again week after week. Non-existent boundaries. Self-loathing. Deep shame. Heavy, drowning guilt. Exhaustion.

A sadness that feels like it penetrates my bones.
At my very core, I feel unworthy.

♥ JO'S TOOLKIT: LESSER-KNOWN SIGNS OF LOW SELF-ESTEEM

▶ Slouching. This could be a sign you're trying to not be seen. A way to retreat inwards, to protect your inner child by taking up as little space as possible.

▶ Saying sorry WAY too much.

▶ Buying things to impress others.

▶ Not being able to take a compliment.

▶ Not being able to make simple decisions.

▶ Giving up easily.

▶ Locked in a cycle of compare and despair.

▶ Not being able to handle criticism.

▶ Twisting yourself in knots to please people, even those you don't like.

▶ Not leaving the house without make-up.

▶ Letting others take the lead.

▶ Retreating from confrontation.

▶ Thinking that anything good in your life is pure luck.

- Compulsively picking your skin or scabs, biting your nails or pulling out your hair/eyelashes/eyebrows.

- Taking more naps than a baby.

- Using your phone as a social prop if alone in public.

I feel exposed.

I feel naked, as if I am literally undressing and unwrapping myself in front of her.

I feel vulnerability and shame in exposing what lies beneath the many curated layers I've so comfortably wrapped myself in for years.

I expect rejection. I expect her to recoil in horror at how fundamentally awful I am. I expect her to be shocked by the cavernous, hollow emptiness inside me.

But it doesn't happen. Instead, I am consistently met time after time with acceptance, understanding, validation and kindness.

When I say I feel like I am treading water, going around and around in the same repeated circles, Elinor reassures me this is normal and that it doesn't matter. In fact, she says that repetition is a positive attribute in therapy because each time I bring up the same topic, I will see it in a slightly different light – new concerns present themselves with new themes. Our brains are like wheat fields. Old pathways are well worn and easy to see and follow. We have to choose the new path again and again before it becomes the easier route to walk. Through the iteration and reiteration of what initially seems like many disconnected branches and roots, it becomes clear they are all intertwined in a single tree.

At an almost imperceptibly slow pace and with each tiny step, each small part of myself I reveal, I feel things start to shift within me.

And not just within me. It slowly starts to dawn on me that my attitude to therapy has changed too. Elinor and therapy have become a consistent, dependable, stable part of my life. My weekly sessions feel like the anchor point to my week. My reset button. A vital part of reclaiming who I am. I'm also surprised to realise that, even though many of my sessions are still very tough, I actually look forward to therapy.

Elinor makes me begin to feel worthy.

Therapy thoughts

Dr Christina Iglesia, licensed clinical psychologist and founder of the #therapyiscool mental health action campaign, tells me, '*One of the most common misconceptions is that the only people who go to or benefit from therapy are those struggling with a mental health condition. In reality, therapy can offer a valuable experience to anyone who is open to it. Therapy is one of the few opportunities in which you are encouraged to explore and express your authentic self, allowing for deeper personal connections and engagement in life. While research states that therapy is the treatment of choice for mental health conditions, it is also an available avenue for personal growth.*'

Chapter Four
THERAPY IS
Eye-opening

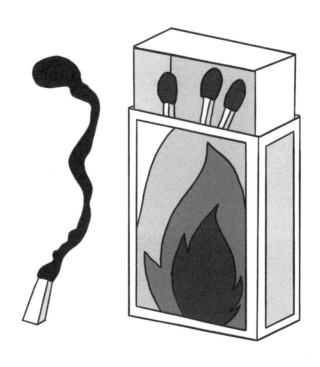

I loved corporate life. And when I say I loved it, I mean I *really* loved it. If you'd have met me during my mid- to late twenties you would have seen this for yourself. You would have seen a successful lawyer, at the top of her game advising some of the world's largest tech giants on cutting-edge and innovative areas of law. It would have looked like I had it all, and for a while I really did.

BURNING OUT

Corporate life satisfyingly scratches my perfectionist itch. My drive to do it all and to do it better is not just shared and understood, it is actively encouraged. For years I find genuine satisfaction in working super long hours, tackling the mountains of paperwork and taking on more and more tight deadlines. I love it all.

And I continue to love it, until I really don't. Because what I won't know until many years later is that this is, in fact, the very worst possible place I could be. Corporate life will wear me down, burn me out, chew me up and eventually destroy me and spit me out without so much as a backwards glance. And as a chronic achiever I am unconsciously complicit in this destruction. I will actively help to build, brick by brick, my unhealthy prison within which I will voluntarily shackle myself and willingly serve my time before my eventual and somewhat abrupt early release, after I have been used up and no longer serve any purpose. I burn the candle at both ends. I work every hour there is, taking on more and more. I ignore the warning signs and push myself to my limit and beyond.

I don't see until it is too late just how used to being burned out I become. How my excuses of 'I need to get through this project and then I'll take a break', 'I'll feel better after the weekend/this holiday', 'I just need to tick off a few more items on my to-do list to ease some pressure' never work. I learn the hard way that burnout doesn't go away on its own and, left unchecked, it can and does brutally break you.

♥ JO'S TOOLKIT: SIGNS OF WORKPLACE BURNOUT

In general, burnout feels just like you'd imagine. Like you've been burned to the ground and all that's left behind are the charred embers and ashes of your life. There is nothing left to give. That said, it can show up in a variety of different ways for different people:

▸ *The spark has gone.* You're unable to muster up enthusiasm for the things that usually energise you – this goes for activities outside the office too.

▸ *You're on a hamster wheel.* It all feels futile. The harder you work, the faster the wheel seems to spin and you can never catch up. You push yourself harder thinking that's the solution, but really you're accelerating faster into burnout.

▸ *You can't be arsed.* Maybe you've found you just can't be as caring, empathetic or compassionate as you usually are to those around you. This apathy, disillusionment and cynicism might also present itself as a dip in performance. Have you started making careless or simple errors, or consistently missing deadlines? If so, it might be a sign you have burnout on your hands.

▶ *Sunday night dread.* Does your heart sink as your alarm goes off each morning? Are you trudging to your desk each day? Not relishing the end of the weekend is a pretty normal feeling, but if the looming shadow of Monday starts to bring with it more anxiety, stress or sadness than normal, it might be a sign of something more sinister.

▶ *You're knackered,* and not in the normal lack of sleep for a couple of nights kinda way. This is more a feeling of being physically and emotionally exhausted all the time, no matter how much rest you seem to have. Weekends are never long enough; time off only provides temporary relief if you're lucky.

▶ *Physical symptoms.* There doesn't seem to be one consistent physical symptom of burnout, but things to watch out for include headaches, chest pains and stomach aches or intestinal issues.

It got to the point where my burnout was so severe anyone just casually asking me how I was would result in me bursting into uncontrollable tears. I had been carrying too much, for too long. I couldn't hold it in anymore, it was like the internal dam that had been holding the mounting tide of pressure back for all these years had finally broken and there was now nothing I could do to repair it. I felt like such a failure, the only lawyer who couldn't hack it. I wasn't tough enough. I wasn't strong enough. I wasn't enough.

Even though it was the right decision, leaving law wasn't an easy thing to do. So much of my life and identity was tied up in being a lawyer. But I did it. I walked away from friends, a community, everything I had worked so hard for and, of course, that lovely big pay packet.

Life on the outside of the glass and steel towers was new

and strange and a little bit scary. But I didn't have long to dwell on it as I quickly found myself with a new business and an even longer to-do list than I had ever had as a lawyer. I ran an online marketplace selling gifts aimed at mums and their small people. It was important to me that the business wasn't just about selling stuff; it needed to have a bigger purpose. And that purpose was one close to my heart – to raise awareness and help mums suffering with mental health issues. The business donated money to charities in this area, hosted events, used its platform to raise awareness in the hope that if I just helped one mum feel a little less alone, my job would be done.

And what a thrill it was; I was at the helm, I held the keys to my own time. I had no boss, no time sheets to fill out, no stuffy corporate office environment, and no more suits! And above all, the business meant something. I wasn't just making money for the corporate machine. In fact, I wasn't making any money at all, but what I was doing was making a difference. Maternal mental health was my passion, my motivation, my new North Star. I had never felt so free.

REPEATING THE CYCLE

Elinor looks me in the eye and I know something I am not going to like is about to come out of her mouth. I can sense it. My insides clench waiting for whatever blow she's about to deal. I feel my jaw stiffen and my insides harden.

Her tone is gentle but serious.

She says she's worried about me and has been for some time. She says she thinks I'm heading towards rock bottom, fast. She says I'm at a critical point. I need to rest, I need to put the brakes on and look after myself.

I don't meet her eye, instead I watch the sunlight on the wall.

'I don't know what you mean,' I say in a small, not very convincing voice.

I know exactly what she means.

I've been at it again; my life has become too much. I've been doing too much. Too much work, too much time on social media, too much presenting a sparkly front to the world, too much time spent responding to strangers' emotional distress at all hours of the day and night, too much putting myself at the bottom of the pile, just too much. I'm repeating the old cycle: recovery, burnout, recovery, burnout. Unknowingly I've taken all the pressures I knew so well in my corporate life and voluntarily recreated them in my new business life. So much for feeling free; here I am feeling trapped yet again. The all-consuming ambition to make it work rages through me – the unrelenting pressure, the long hours, the lack of sleep, the pushing my body and mind to the edge. All so familiar to me, all so toxic. But this time there is no boss breathing down my neck, no competitive office culture, nope... this time I have no one to blame but myself.

I feel very, very stretched, so thin I think I might almost snap.

Elinor softly but firmly continues: 'If you had a normal job, I'd be recommending that you were signed off work again, but since you have a business to run how would it feel if you took some time off social media?'

That's when the severity of the situation hits me.

Oh God, she is right. I know something needs to change. I know I am not well.

The familiar feelings of depression and running on empty, that for weeks have been humming unnoticed under the surface, are now so blindingly obvious. It's as if Elinor has shined her torch into my darkness and shown me what is there. Now I can't un-see it.

No sooner have these thoughts formed than my brain snaps into defence mode.

I don't want to see, I want to un-see.

Time off? Is she mad? It's impossible. She doesn't understand how it all works, I rationalise to myself. She's older, she's only on Facebook recreationally, she doesn't get how this dynamic fast-paced world of social media marketing works.

'Nope, I'm sorry but that's not going to be possible,' I bluster, not wanting to look her in the eye. 'You see, I need to be on social media. I... I have to be there.'

I feel a bit desperate now and possibly as if I'm pleading with her. Am I pleading with her? I can feel the rawness of fear catch in my throat. Oh God, I *am* pleading with her. I ignore it and push on.

'You see, any time away, even just for a day and my engagement will drop,' I say matter of factly, 'and that cannot happen, because then the algorithm will punish me.' I'm sounding a bit paranoid now. I can hear it and so can she. I see it on her face. But I keep going: 'My business will suffer.'

I notice my voice is starting to take on a screeching edge. I take a deep breath and calm myself before delivering what I think is a killer blow to her argument: 'And that will be even more detrimental to my mental health.'

Aha. I've got her. Check bloody mate.

Silence.

There is no joy in this empty victory. Why is there no joy? I should be feeling triumphant for this nifty piece of mental manoeuvring.

More silence.

Why is she still looking at me?

But see, that's the thing, she doesn't need to say anything. I can feel her thoughts percolate into me regardless.

Gah, I know she is right.

More silence.

My thoughts race around and around on a loop. I want a break, I need a break, but I can't. I want a break, I need a break, but I can't. I am trapped. There is no choice.

More silence.

'OK, OK, you're right,' I begrudgingly concede. 'But help me do this,' I say.

I am falling apart, I need help. I am spiralling downwards fast yet again, and the bottom feels frighteningly close. But this time it feels different, this time Elinor is my early warning system, jolting me into a wake-up call. This time I have Elinor. I am not alone.

Together we sit in the dark, her light giving the support and hope I so desperately need. Together we tackle this.

We go through a list of pros and cons, which I write on my phone so I can look at it when I leave the session. I still have that list today. Looking at it, it's pretty obvious what I need to do. I need to press pause. I need to rest.

I leave my session having very reluctantly agreed to try a social media break of one week, and if I'm honest I only do this because that's what I think is the minimum Elinor will let me get away with. And if I'm really laying it bare, I don't think I will be able to do it, and realise I've already started concocting various excuses in my head.

And it doesn't start well as I don't start my switch-off immediately.

First, I have to go to a festival in Oxfordshire where, at an astronomical cost I can barely afford at a time when my business, which had now been going for a couple of years at this point, is

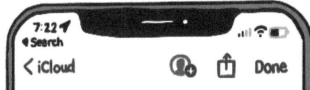

7:22
◀ Search

‹ iCloud

Pros

I'm burned out, running on empty,
I need a break

Yearning for balance, my family life
is suffering

My own MH is suffering

Craving connection with people in
the real world

Want to stop filling every spare moment
thinking about social media

Want to stop the compare and
despair trap

Need to regain space and time to
heal

Cons

Potential impact on sales

The algorithm might punish me
when I return

People might forget me/the business

on a knife edge of make or break. I have a stall selling some of our stock. I justify to myself the whole shebang will need to be documented on social media and therefore I have to keep going, just for one more long weekend anyway.

It's the end of August and after a blisteringly hot summer with what feels like not a drop of rain since May, the heavens open and there is no let-up for the entire weekend. It rains continuously, from the moment I set foot out of my house until the festival is eventually shut down prematurely three days later due to the inclement conditions.

It rains throughout the four hours I am left immovable on an M25 slip road on the way there. No turning around, not able to move an inch backwards or forwards. If ever there was a metaphor for my life right now, this is bloody it.

I.

Am.

Stuck.

And the list of catastrophes goes on and on – you honestly couldn't make it up. My tent leaks every night, meaning each morning I wake up in a cold soggy puddle. The sales are abysmal, the weekend a disaster in every sense of the word. To add insult to injury, my car has a puncture on the way home, and the roof box bursts open, spewing my stock as well as the remaining parts of my sanity with it all over the road.

The entire weekend feels like I am in a vortex of negativity. I am in a vicious cycle being sucked downwards and there is nothing I can do to stop the spiral of decline. It is the nail in the coffin for the business too, as somewhere in the midst of this soggy miserable mess I make the decision that by the end of the year I need to close the website down. I feel yet again like such a failure, but the figures don't add up and my heart is just not in retail – my motivation is maternal mental health, not being a salesperson. But how can I shout about mental health when I can't even look after my own right now? I realise the irony of this at the time. Something feels very wrong, and something needs to change.

I get home and I collapse. Literally and metaphorically. I need a break, because I am broken open.

I reach for my phone and delete my social media apps. I can't do it anymore, I'm done.

♥ JO'S TOOLKIT: SIGNS YOU MIGHT NEED A DIGITAL DETOX

▶ Your phone is the first thing you reach for when you wake up and the last thing you touch before you sleep.

▶ Managing your social media account is starting to feel like a full-time job.

▶ You get twitchy if you're separated from your phone.

▶ Losing your phone feels like a legitimate reason for a breakdown.

▶ You regularly fall down the rabbit hole of scrolling random accounts without any recollection of how or why you got there.

▶ You check, check and re-check your phone for new social media notifications.

▶ The number of likes or comments you get really affects whether you're bummed out or in a great mood.

▶ You can't stop comparing your life to the picture-perfect curated social feeds of others.

▶ Screen time is your only down time.

RISING FROM THE ASHES

Recovering from burnout is a long, slow road and avoiding it now feels like a lifelong challenge. Therapy helped me see what wasn't right in my working life and identify what was causing me to keep repeating the cycle and playing with fire. It gave me practical coping strategies for fighting the flames as well as helping me fireproof myself by slowing me down and giving me healthier ways of navigating life's stresses.

Learning how to recover from burnout will look different to different people as there can be many different causes, many ways it shows up and many more ways to get rid of it.

For me, social media had taken over my every waking moment. A quick post while standing in the queue waiting for the bus, in between loading the dishwasher, in the semi darkness, the blue light of my phone glowing, waiting for Bella to fall asleep, my brain always whirring thinking of content, answering direct messages, responding to comments, feeling the pressure to keep showing up, posting, giving, liking, sharing, responding to hundreds and hundreds of messages. Meaning my initially reluctant week-long break turned into me voluntarily taking many months away from scrolling, giving me some much-needed space to breathe again.

My burnout also stems from my self-imposed pressure to always perform flawlessly. In short, my need to be perfect.

Meaning, for me, there is no instant cure from burnout as no amount of rest, sleep, self-care or mindfulness can take away my perfectionism. But therapy has allowed me to reframe my thoughts, including how to say no, how to have boundaries and how to know when to switch off.

LEARNING HOW TO SAY NO

Two little letters. One small syllable. One word, but also an entire sentence. Something so small, but something I find almost impossible to utter.

I've never been good at saying no. Instead I am a habitual yesser. I comply, I please, I agree. I am a yes girl.

But scratch the surface and being a yes girl is not quite so wonderful; the life of a yes girl actually has some pretty big drawbacks.

The problem is that I say yes to everyone and everything.

I say yes to more work when I really need to rest, meaning in the past I have walked into the office on Wednesday morning and not left until late Friday night. When I'm asked on the street if I'd like to take part in a survey, I say yes, when I'm already running late. I say yes to favours from so-called friends who only moments earlier have been deeply offensive to me. I've found myself in scary and dangerous situations because I've been too polite to speak up. I've been on dates with people I have had zero interest in. I've paid for botched hairdos and left with a smile rather than a complaint.

The list goes on and on.

But somewhere along the way, therapy has helped me see that by doing this I'm not quite living my life. Instead, I seem to have created a schedule that is a strange combination of mainly meeting the expectations of others, a fair bit of what I think I should be doing and only a tiny sliver of what I actually want to do. The result? I have a never-ending to-do list that often leaves me overwhelmed and unfulfilled. I go to events I don't want to go to; I buy things I don't want to buy; I hang out with people I don't like; I go for a drink when I decided I was going to stay sober that week; I am chronically overbooked and overwhelmed. Yes so often feels easier than no – no is obstructive, no is awkward, no could hurt or insult, no is rude. I really don't want to disappoint people, I don't want to let them down.

And Elinor sees this is what I've done too.

She helps me to identify that swapping law for the entrepreneurial life, far from being the expected release, in reality did very little for my inability to say no. In fact, if anything, it only exacerbated my need to take on more and lessen my ability to switch off. At the same time, motherhood was taking its toll with my need to do it all, be it all. And my social life was no different, the product of years of finding myself sucked into a succession of toxic power dynamics of various 'queen bees' who I so desperately wanted to be liked and accepted by, but who I couldn't stand up to, wouldn't dare say no to, and who in reality actually made me increasingly miserable and worn down.

My therapist says, 'I have a theory, which may be a little simplistic, but I think it works. I think there are largely two types of people in the world, Jo. There are the takers and then there are the givers. Takers put their own interests ahead of others' needs. They are not necessarily bad people, but they do naturally try to gain as much as possible from their interactions while contributing as little as they can in return. Givers, on the other hand, are focused on others and tend to provide support to others with no strings attached, but often to their own detriment.

'You are a giver, and you have unknowingly surrounded

yourself with takers. This isn't your fault; it's what you are drawn to, because this is what you've always known.'

This certainly seems to ring true.

And it's what she says next that really hits home.

'It's completely OK to say no to a taker. The vast majority of takers will not take your no personally. They will expect the no, they're used to hearing no. If you find it helpful, think of it as if they're waiting for the no. They ask, they hear no, they will move on to ask someone else. And they will assume that if you've said yes it's because you want to do it. They will think to themselves, "She wouldn't have agreed to this if she didn't want to do it, she would have just said no." No is an easy word for them. It is as simple as black and white: you want to do it, you'll agree; you don't, then you'll say no. They won't understand that you are saying yes because you fear rejection, don't want to disappoint, make them angry, hurt their feelings or appear unkind or rude... or any of the other reasons you find it so hard to say no.'

Aha. This makes so much sense.

JO'S TOOLKIT: MY THREE TINY TIPS FOR SAYING NO

1   *Stop elaborating*. Too often, I over-explain myself into a corner. My default tends to be, 'Oh, I'm so sorry, I have another thing that day, and it probably won't end in time, though I guess there's a chance it will finish early, and if it does, then maybe I can...' and then I end up doing the thing I didn't want to, on top of everything else. I've got to get better at 'I'm sorry, I won't be able to make it' and then shutting the hell up.

2   *Stop apologising*. OK, so there are definitely times I do need to say sorry for things, but if sorry becomes too extreme a habit, then we can start convincing ourselves we are doing something wrong by setting normal healthy limits. 'I can't take that on right now, but I hope you're able to find someone' is a good alternative to 'sorry I can't do that' at work.

3   *Suggest an alternative*. 'It's such a shame I'll have to miss your party. But can I take you out to lunch sometime instead?' But of course, this is only to be used if you do actually want to do the alternative!

The fallout from saying no is never as bad as I think it will be. The sky doesn't fall, the world doesn't stop turning, my family don't stop loving me, my friends don't stop liking me, and almost everyone probably respects me and my time more.

It might be useful to share with you some of the ways this self-confessed 'people-pleasing nice girl' has learned through therapy to say no minus the guilt. One day I hope to be able to utter with confidence the straight 'No, thank you', but while I work on that one, I've found this list handy to wriggle myself more comfortably out of things:

▶ 'I'm going to pass this time, but thank you for thinking of me.'

▶ 'That sounds great, but it hasn't come at a good time for me.'

▶ 'Thanks for inviting me/asking me, sadly I can't this time.'

▶ 'I've been taking on too much recently, so I'm going to have to pass.'

▶ 'I promised myself I would carve out some time to switch off, so it means I can't this time.'

▶ 'I'd love to hang out/go for drinks/do that thing, but I really need to rest.'

▶ 'Can we look at doing this later in the week/month/year?' (Trust me, only use this strategy if you mean it, because people do come back to you!)

And sometimes if you're not immediately sure if you want to say yes or no, create a pause instead by saying:

▶ 'Why don't we talk about this next week/next month/later in the year?'

- ❭ 'Let me reflect on that and get back to you.'

- ❭ 'I don't have an answer right now, but I will let you know.'

- ❭ 'I need to take a moment to mull that over.'

HOW TO HAVE BOUNDARIES

Like saying the word no, I have struggled and still struggle with creating, maintaining and enforcing personal boundaries in all areas of my life.

But what exactly are boundaries? I see them as the invisible emotional lines I won't allow others to cross. They are less about keeping myself separate from others, and more about the ways in which I will connect. My boundaries are a way of telling people, 'Hey! This is how you can treat me, and this is how you cannot treat me.' They act like fences we create between ourselves and the outside world. We all have them, but just how strong or high those fences are will vary from person to person.

'But I just can't,' I practically wail at Elinor when she gently suggests for the umpteenth time that it might be useful to firm up some of my boundaries with some people in my life. 'I just can't do it. It's too awkward. Plus, people will think I'm rude... I'd be letting people down, it all feels far too selfish.'

'I hear you. But can I give you an example of one of my boundaries that might help?'

I nod mutely.

'Staying within our 50-minute session here in therapy is a boundary I need to keep to. If I didn't, I would spend hours and hours with each client, letting my later clients down by running over, but also exhausting myself mentally and physically in the process. When we start to approach the end of our time together and I say something like, "We are coming to the end of our time today, let's pick this up again next week", is it awkward or do you think I'm being rude? Do you think I've let you down? Does it feel like I'm being selfish? Have you even noticed it as a boundary?'

'Er, well, no. Sure, sometimes I'd like longer with you and that's occasionally frustrating, but I know that we can't go on all day. I do respect that. I get that the line needs to be drawn somewhere and, thinking about it, it's actually a relief you're in charge of that one. I really value the time we do have.'

'Uh-huh. And did you notice the words you used there? "Respect", "value", "relief" and "in charge", which really couldn't be further from "awkward", "selfish" and "rude" could they?'

She has a point.

♥ JO'S TOOLKIT: MY TOP TIPS ON BOUNDARIES

▶ Try as much as humanly possible to communicate your boundaries to those you want to respect them. When doing so, use as few words as possible. Never apologise. Never justify yourself or over-explain.

▶ Remember, having boundaries is hard and takes practice – the boundary-setting muscle takes time to develop.

▶ Starting small and practising with strangers you'll never see again might help.

▶ You can, and will, feel any combination of guilt, selfishness and embarrassment about setting, maintaining and enforcing boundaries. Remember this is normal.

▶ Most people won't even notice you've set a boundary. That said, there will always be some people who will never accept your boundaries whatever you do or say. It says more about them than you. Try to remain firm.

▶ You can, and very often should, have different boundaries with different people; boundaries are not a one-size-fits-all solution.

▶ Boundaries are not barriers or shutters to the world. I personally need to remember this and to lower my emotional walls at times in order to let some of the positive experiences in, like accepting compliments or allowing others to help me once in a while.

▶ Resentment, exhaustion or frequent moaning are often red flags for needing to put a boundary in place (or giving an existing one a tweak).

▶ The ink isn't permanent. Boundaries should be flexible – they are not another stick to beat yourself with. Be careful not to set them too high and remember to revisit them when needed.

People who care about you will respect your boundaries and adapt. However, sometimes those closest to us can be the most stubborn about adjusting to the new versions of ourselves. They might think they know what's best for us, steamrolling right through our attempts at boundaries. When you can't keep them at arm's length because maybe you live with them or your lives are too intertwined, my tip would be to stay alert around them, keep it kind and keep it consistent, i.e. 'You know how much I love you, but I told you I have it under control. I know it's hard, but please respect this. When I do need your help, I promise I'll reach out.' I also find it helpful to get my mental highlighter pen out and mark their name with fluorescent ink, flagging them as 'boundary pushers' and people to watch myself around.

Some of my boundaries be like...

▶ I do not have to respond immediately to a text, WhatsApp, social media message or email.

▶ Very few people in my life are owed or need an explanation for my decisions.

▶ I'm allowed to take time off.

▶ It is not my job to make everyone around me happy.

▶ It's OK if people don't like me.

▶ It's OK if I don't like certain people.

▶ I do not have to feel guilty for standing up for myself.

▶ I do not have to feel guilty for liking myself.

▶ It's OK to say 'That isn't something I want to talk about.'

▶ It's OK to say 'I don't agree with that, and I don't want to be a part of it.'

▶ It's OK for someone to be part of your past but not part of your future.

I'm still not there with feeling wholly comfortable with saying no and creating boundaries, but I've found therapy has definitely helped me identify the not-so-obvious takers in my life. It has also given me the strength and courage to change a few of those endless yesses into nos.

Therapy thoughts

When writing this book I reached out to Elinor to get her honest take on all things therapy. Here's what she told me when I asked her whether there were any common themes that clients struggle with: 'Clients often have low self-compassion, their internal voice can be really mean and judgemental. This can often lead to a fear of judgement from others. Another common theme is boundaries, both in work and private life. Mental health is as important as physical health and creating balance and boundaries is vital.'

Chapter Five
THERAPY IS
A Privilege

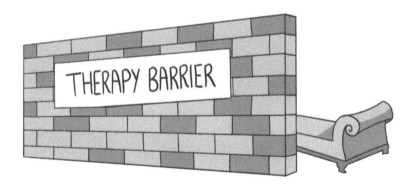

While there are multiple barriers to entry for mental health treatment, such as lack of professionals or services, lack of awareness, lack of childcare, perceived lack of spare time, travel problems, doubts about the need for help, the prevalence of stigma, cultural, religious or spiritual attitudes, disparities in mental health care access among different racial and ethnic groups and the reluctance to talk about personal issues, the high cost is often a major factor in why people don't access mental health care.

I've been quietly stewing on this issue for some time now, and well before I had even conceived of this book, I asked my audience on Instagram what their main barriers were to having regular therapy. I wasn't in the least bit surprised to hear the overwhelming majority of people said the cost.

THERAPY IS EXPENSIVE

Before I know it, my allotted six insurance sessions have run out, but I don't feel ready to stop. I feel like the work is only just starting. But it feels like a huge commitment to start paying for therapy and, even though I can see the benefit it is having in so many areas of my life, I still find this an incredibly hard decision to make.

I don't have a stable income, but I am lucky – I have a roof over my head and food in my tummy. Difficult decisions need to be made and the sacrifices feel boring and constant – walking instead of spending money on public transport, deleting shopping apps from my phone, bringing a coffee or my lunch with me rather than buying on the go.

But whenever that pesky little voice pops into my head telling me I can't afford to continue therapy, another one responds to say

MYTHS ABOUT PAYING FOR THERAPY

Myth: 'They are only listening to you because you pay them to.'
Truth: The fact your therapist earns a living by talking to you doesn't mean they don't care about you.

Myth: 'There is no value in therapy; you don't get anything tangible or measurable.'
Truth: We live in a society where material goods are often equated with personal worth and happiness, so we can be forgiven for wondering about the value of spending money on therapy. However, good therapy has the potential to improve our lives far more than we could ever imagine, which is arguably more valuable than having the most Instagrammable outfit, holiday, car, wallpaper, sink, coffee, etc.

Myth: 'It is selfish to spend money on something that only benefits you.'
Truth: It's true that at first it seems as if therapy is all about 'me, me, me', but this simply isn't true – it doesn't just benefit the person sat on the therapist's couch. The changes that we make in our lives as a result of good therapy can and do have a positive ripple effect on how we interact with the world around us, meaning therapy benefits many others in our lives as well.

I can't afford *not* to. Yes, it feels uncomfortable, but it also feels a non-negotiable necessary investment to rebuild myself because I take my mental health and well-being seriously.

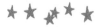

As Clare Seal, author of *Real Life Money* (and aka @MyFrugalYear on Instagram), explains, 'money and mental health are so tightly knitted together for most people that it's almost impossible to consider one without the other interrupting – whether it's the wave of anxiety that hits you when you go to check you bank balance or the financial hit you take when your mental health declines, especially if you're prone to spending as a way to alleviate low mood.

'For a very long time, I was stuck in a never-ending cycle of money and mental health troubles, one perpetuating the other until I decided that I needed help. I knew that I had to tackle both in order to improve either one, but I was worried about the cost of therapy. Initially, I was able to access some free sessions through the NHS, which gave me the boost that I needed to bounce that spiral back in the opposite direction. A couple of years on, both my finances and my mental health are much better as a baseline, and I'm more sensitive to the signs that mean that I need to focus more on either one. When I started to feel depressed during the first wave of the COVID-19 pandemic, my work suffered immediately, and I knew that I needed to reach out again or face another financial hit.

'Now that I know the value of therapy, and its role in keeping my financial and mental well-being in check, I will include it in my budget for as long as I can possibly afford to. Especially as a self-employed person, I can't afford to take weeks off work to try to fix my broken brain again. To me, therapy is as essential as most other things.'

THE COST OF THERAPY

It feels like this should be a place to break out and give you some handy tips on how to budget to afford therapy, but that is condescending and patronising, not to mention it assumes people are in a position to be able to budget or save. Many are not. If this is you, please see Chapter Ten (pages 201 and 202) where not only do I explore some of the lesser known low-cost and free options out there, but also offer some ideas on how to practise self-support responsibly.

In some respects, here in the UK we are luckier than a lot of countries in that there are many mental health services available through the NHS for free. But like everything in life, nothing comes for free without a catch. The main one for most people being that, depending on where you live, it's more than likely you will join a very long waiting list to get access to any of these services. In addition, the therapy on offer will likely differ in different parts of the country and will often be short-term only, normally from around 6 to 12 sessions. It will, of course, depend on why you are going for therapy, but you are unlikely to have much choice on the type you receive and, for a great many people, it is likely to involve CBT, which won't be suitable for everyone. There is more on how to access NHS resources, as well as a number of other services and organisations out there trying to make therapy more accessible to a wider range of people, in Chapter Ten.

If you choose to go down the private route, there will be differences in price depending on the type of therapy you have (some very niche or specialised therapies will cost more), the therapist you see (very experienced therapists generally cost more than those newly qualified or still in training, and psychotherapists will usually be more expensive than counsellors), where you are in the country (for example, in London you can expect a higher price point than in other parts of the country) and, of course, how long you see the therapist for.

When I reached out to my audience on social media, I also asked them what the maximum amount they might be able to afford for weekly therapy was. I then asked a few professionals, including a well-known therapy booking platform, Harley Therapy, to tell me what costs actually are. Interestingly, what people would be prepared to pay versus the average cost were not actually so far apart.

The maximum average people said they would pay was just shy of £40 per hour. At the time of writing, the lowest fees listed on Harley Therapy are £25, with plenty offering sessions at the £30–£45 mark, and the average cost across all their 500 active therapists and therapies was just shy of £60 per session. If it's a helpful indicator, I've paid for therapy with both counsellors and psychotherapists both in and outside London and have always paid in the £40–£50 per hour bracket.

However, the very real truth is that paying for therapy privately, even with the best budgeting skills and prioritisation, is off the cards for many people who would benefit enormously if it was available to them.

RACE AND CULTURE AS A BARRIER TO ENTRY

As we've seen, the cost of therapy can be a huge barrier to entry in someone seeking support. Another big obstacle for many is the issue of race or culture in the therapy experience.

There is a lot to unpack here, but essentially there's no denying that therapy comes from a white, patriarchal system. Generally speaking, white men have for hundreds of years been thinking and writing theories that are then read and taught by other white people, and then applied to more predominately white people.

Therefore, it follows that sometimes some of these models may be unhelpful at best and harmful at worst to non-white people. For example, as Dr Emma Svanberg pointed out to me: 'if someone comes to therapy because they have experienced systemic racism, and the therapist asks them to think about how their behaviours or thoughts might be contributing to their feelings, that in essence is a denial of their lived reality and colludes with the idea they might be responsible for their distress'.

I don't think this is to say a white therapist could never help a Black, Asian and minority ethnic (BAME) client; however there is clearly a growing desire for many to have a therapeutic experience that feels safe and inclusive to their own culture, religion or belief system.

We also know that people from BAME communities are at greater risk of developing mental health conditions than their white counterparts. And despite the increased need for support, a review in 2018 found profound inequalities for BAME individuals seeking, accessing and experiencing mental health services. Another 2013 report found that only 10 per cent of the BAME people surveyed felt that their talking therapy service adequately took into consideration their cultural background, and a third believed that the service was not fit for BAME people.

From the Other Chair
CULTURAL DIFFERENCES

Dr Tina Mistry, clinical psychologist (aka @brownpsychologist on Instagram), says, 'Our histories are full of trauma, loss and pain. However, for many of us, we have had to put that at the back of our minds and do our best to survive in the UK. These erased histories and negative experiences are the make-up of our thoughts, feelings, behaviour, as individuals but also as communities. Therefore, in order for things to change, we need to be seen, I mean really seen and heard. This will include taking into account what our culture deems as healing. So, for many communities talking is not enough or just not the way we do things. Many will use movement, art, music, narrative, nutrition, connection to religion or spirituality to heal. And when we are the co-designers or creators of services that take into consideration our socio-historical–spiritual perspectives, we may just feel that we are being seen and heard. You don't need to guess what we need; you need to give us a seat at the table where decisions are made so we can tell you.

It might be naïve, but I dream of a Utopian world where everyone could easily and quickly access the correct care and support for them, at zero or very low cost, whenever they wanted and for as long as they needed. Anyone experiencing a mental health concern should be able to confidently know they have speedy access, within an assured timeframe, to effective, tailored care as close to where they live as possible. To know they won't be turned away because of their perceived level of illness, their postcode, their skin colour, their age, their level of income or any other characteristic. And everyone would have the ability to access a variety of talking therapies so that they can pick the one most suitable for them.

I'm certain there is a clever economic model out there that could fully work through the cost–benefit analysis, but I can't help but feel on a gut level it makes sense. When you weigh the cost of mental ill health on the economy, our healthcare system and society – estimated at £105 billion a year in 2015 – against the indisputable benefits therapy has on both mental and physical health, it feels obvious it would save money in both the short and long term on not just mental and physical health provision in the UK, but also the wider economic and social costs too (such as social care services, welfare benefits, lost productivity due to sickness absence, and lost productivity and working hours due to people with mental health problems not being in work).

Maybe this is too simplistic, but in my mind at least, it's not much to ask for mental health to be treated with the same degree of seriousness as physical health. After all, in the end, it all adds to our public and private well-being.

Therapy thoughts

'Black people deserve access to therapeutic services and mental health support that takes into account the specific issues that come up when accessing Eurocentric models of mental health. These are issues such as language, and cultural and traditional barriers.'

Agnes Mwakatuma, founder of the charity Black Minds Matter

Chapter Six
THERAPY IS
Hard

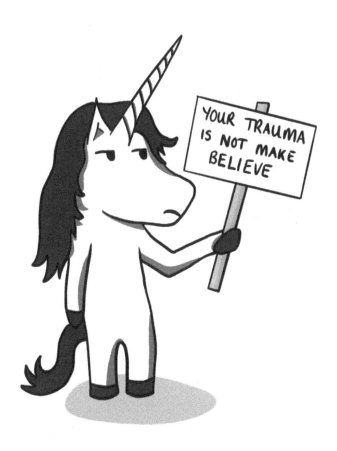

'I think you have PTSD,' Elinor says softly after I've been telling her about yet another panic attack I've had recently. 'What you're describing to me are what are known as triggers.

'Triggers operate on a subconscious level so you won't be able to just will them away. There are things we can do together to help you manage them, but ongoing vigilance like this, that never rests, is exhausting, so instead let's try to free you of them altogether.'

I scrunch my face at her and think to myself, 'That's not possible, I can't have PTSD. That's reserved for battlefields or near-death experiences, not from mental illnesses themselves.'

She reads my scepticism and says, 'Trauma can be caused by any traumatic experience, not just an assault or natural disaster; it can be caused by the intense emotional distress you felt during your maternal mental illness.'

I'm in shock. This is all completely new information to me.

She goes on to explain: 'Traumatic memories live in our brains differently to usual memories. Our ordinary memories slot neatly into our life narratives; they have a place, time and context, and stand out only if they were particularly emotionally charged, like one or two standout photos in a chronologically-ordered album.' But she tells me: 'Traumatic memories are stored differently. They're lessons our brains learn to help protect us from future threats.'

'Ah,' I say, 'like fight, flight or freeze?'

'Yes, exactly.' She looks pleased with me and I predictably flush with pride.

'But it's like your "fight, flight or freeze" button has got stuck in the switched-on position.'

From the Other Chair
POST-TRAUMATIC STRESS DISORDER (PTSD)

As Laura Bethel (@cotswoldemdr on Instagram), psycho-therapist and EMDR specialist, explains, PTSD is a type of anxiety disorder that you may develop after being involved in, or witnessing, traumatic events. The condition was first recognised in war veterans and has been known by a variety of names, such as 'shell shock', 'combat fatigue' and 'soldier's heart'. But it's not only diagnosed in soldiers – there are a wide range of traumatic experiences that can cause PTSD symptoms, whether that's a car accident, a rocky childhood, witnessing or being involved in a violent assault, childbirth, a medical complication or diagnosis, a sudden death in the family or a stressful divorce. When lots of incidents are linked it leads to 'complex PTSD'.

Someone with PTSD often relives the traumatic event through dreams or memories, and may experience feelings of isolation, irritability and guilt. They may also have problems sleeping, such as insomnia, and find concentrating difficult. These symptoms are often severe and persistent enough to have a significant impact on the person's day-to-day life.

Symptoms usually develop immediately after someone experiences a traumatic experience. This is a normal part of the way our brains process events and not everyone who experiences trauma will develop PTSD. When a memory does not get properly processed, symptoms can persist for weeks, months or even years, often leading to avoidance and depression.

Triggers

A trigger in psychology is a stimulus, such as a smell, sound or sight, that triggers feelings of trauma. People typically use this term when describing PTSD.

A trigger is a reminder of a past trauma. This reminder can cause a person to feel overwhelming sadness, shame, anxiety or panic. It may also cause someone to have flashbacks. A flashback is a vivid, often negative, memory that may appear without warning. It can cause someone to lose track of their surroundings and dissociate or 'relive' a traumatic event.

Triggers can take many forms. They may be a physical location or the anniversary of the traumatic event. A person could also be triggered by internal processes such as stress or pain.

Sometimes triggers are predictable. For instance, those who have been in combat may have flashbacks while watching a violent movie. In other cases, triggers are less intuitive. A person who smelled incense during a sexual assault may have a panic attack when they smell the same incense in a shop.

CLEARING THE LANDSLIDE

'Think about the traumatic memories as if they are landslides on the road of your life,' Elinor says. 'Your mind can no longer follow the same path it did before. Sure, you can go around these hurdles, which is what you're trying to do right now when you're not frozen, but those routes are bumpy, long and uncomfortable. Let's work together on clearing the landslides and smoothing your road. Let's do EMDR.'

EMDR therapy is a psychotherapy technique that utilises

sensory input such as eye movements to help people recover from trauma (see page 192). At my next session with Elinor there is a tripod set up in the room with what looks like a spirit level attached to the top of it. Elinor flicks a switch and it lights up. Little rectangles of moving blue light appear, which I track across the light bar with my eyes. An eighties reference here, but it looks exactly like the light on the front of KITT, the talking car from the TV programme *Knight Rider*, except it is blue not red.

I'm nervous, but I try to relax and let my eyes follow the light.

Left and then right. Back and forth.

My chest tightens as I picture the day I unravel about Chris's run. I'm watching the room in freeze-frame, like someone has pressed the pause button. My emotions are at their peak. I'm sitting on the bed, Chris is by the window, Bella asleep in her cot. No one is moving. The image is static but it's in 3D. If I wanted to I could walk around that small blue bedroom, peek into cupboards, look under the bed, see it and all its participants from all angles, *Matrix*-style or like a virtual reality video game.

'How distressed are you now, from one to ten, when you think about that day?'

'Nine, this feels like I'm back there. Definitely nine.'

Left, right. Backwards, forwards.

And soon, within that therapy room and my chest, something bubbles up. My whole body locks and trembles. Without warning, tears begin streaming from my eyes. My breath grows sharp and off-tempo. I am back. I am feeling the pain all over again, the anger is not simmering, it's boiling inside of me, and at the same time I am drowning in helplessness and despair.

She stops the light and tells me to take a big breath. I do.

She asks, 'What comes up?', which will be the catchphrase of my EMDR.

I describe the pain.

We go again. Left, right.

The tears come immediately this time, breath instantly ragged.

Somehow there's something bigger within me and it rises without my control. I feel my mouth open and my teeth clench. It's completely sensory, I hear it and feel it all as if I'm someone else, spectating my own pain. I can feel a deep, tight knot of fear, anger, anxiety and loathing deep in the pit of me. Suffocating, asphyxiating guilt. It feels horrible. It astounds me.

Stop.

Big breath.

'What comes up?'

I describe the physical sensations.

We go again. Left, and right.

Again and again we do this.

Again and again I face the visceral feelings inside my body and my mind, over and over. I dread her starting the light each time. I dread the emotions returning.

Stop.

Big breath.

'What comes up?'

This time, they are less strong, but still worth fearing. I clutch two tissues in one fist, waiting, dreading.

I am kicking that landslide, rolling boulder by boulder out of my path. This is so fucking hard.

Stop.

Big breath.

'What comes up?'

Less, everything is just a little less: still present, but not quite so terrifying. Still painful, but not destructive.

Round and round we go again, until eventually...

'What comes up?'

Nothing much, I feel neutral.

'How distressed are you now, from one to ten, when you think about that day?'

'One or two,' I reply, stunned at my answer. 'Though I feel sad about that time still, so there might be some residual sadness.' I can remember the feelings, I can picture the room, I know how hurt I feel, but I feel distanced from it. The rawness and heat has been calmed and cooled.

We take five minutes to calm down before I go home. We meditate, we go to my safe space. I decompress. But my body is limp like a rag doll, and I'm covered in tears and a fair bit of snot. Walking out of her garden office back up the path and into my car feels like it takes my very last ounce of strength. I sit in my car and cry. Silent, dry, heaving tears of someone who has no more tears left inside. I go home and curl up and don't move for the rest of the day.

THERAPY HANGOVERS

Something no one tells you about is the therapy hangovers. Well, they didn't tell me anyway.

This is the term I use to describe the emotional crash that often shows up after I've had a particularly heavy, difficult or intense session. But don't be lulled into a false sense of security by that description; rather annoyingly, they can also appear after seemingly lighter sessions. There is no pattern that I have managed to decipher. In fact, as I type, I'm currently battling a therapy hangover that descended following possibly one of the lightest chit-chat-type sessions I've had in a long while. Go figure! Typically, these hangovers usually last anywhere from a few hours up to a few days following an intense or difficult session. Very occasionally, they can last most of the week between sessions.

My most intense and regular therapy hangovers were always after my EMDR sessions. I would leave with very strict instructions from Elinor to go home, not to work for the rest of the day and sit on the sofa watching one of her personal favourites, *RuPaul's Drag Race*, on repeat. Often with the added suggestion to buy myself a giant chocolate bar on the way home, just to make the experience extra comforting!

WHAT THERAPY HANGOVERS FEEL LIKE

For me, therapy hangovers can be different each time, but the main feeling is like the emotional bus has not just run me over, but someone stuck it in reverse and mowed me down again just to make sure the job had been done. It is the intense urge to retreat from the world and lick my wounds. It is the feeling of being zapped of all energy, wanting to melt into a puddle on the sofa and wrap myself in a duvet cocoon in an attempt to recharge. Post-therapy I've felt everything from a bit 'meh', shaken, upset and anxious to feeling suddenly really stressed, very reactive, tense, shattered and totally drained, along with more physical feelings, such as a bad tummy and feeling a bit tender.

In an ideal world, we would all just hibernate for as long as it takes for us to start to feel better, but in reality, after the hour we've already set aside for the therapy session itself, as well as any travel to and from our appointment, there is no extra time in our lives to allocate to decompression. That said, I've found it helpful to try to keep a relatively clear schedule post-therapy sessions, but when that's not possible, I rearrange my day a little so I'm not immediately tasked with something incredibly taxing.

♥ JO'S TOOLKIT: HOW TO RECOVER FROM A THERAPY HANGOVER

If I do need to jump straight into something, I've discovered some tiny practices that can help:

▶ *Sit quietly* afterwards with your thoughts, even if it's just for five minutes with your phone off. Spend a moment noticing what you are feeling and remind yourself that thoughts are not facts.

▶ If you don't even have five minutes, *take a deep breath* and have a moment to pause.

▶ *Practise mindfulness.* I like the little grounding exercise on page 23. I often get the order muddled but it still works to calm me down!

▶ *Jot it down.* It helps if I note down a few thoughts immediately after my session; normally this is just on my phone. Anything positive or affirming your therapist said, jot it down. Those gems have a way of slipping from our grasp all too easily. Look at them the next day or as often as you need.

▶ *Reframe the fatigue.* This is a tough one, but thinking about the feelings of discomfort or exhaustion as a sign of progress or of better times ahead can be enormously helpful.

▶ Find a way to *connect with your body physically.* Sing, dance, wiggle, have a good long stretch, do five minutes of yoga, massage a tense part of you, hug someone, a pet or a cushion!

▶ *Go for a walk.* Look at what's around you, notice the smells, listen to the sounds. Just five minutes with nature has been proven to have hugely calming and mood-boosting effects.

▶ *Sketch it out.* Well worth a try, even if art isn't your thing. Quickly sketching an analogy of the session can really help process your feelings. What would this session look like if it were an animal or an inanimate object? If you do happen to have paints or coloured pens handy, play with what colour the session might have.

▶ *Rest.* Because it takes hard work to grow.

THERAPY IS HARD WORK

Even when things in therapy are going relatively smoothly, it's rarely an easy process. It is hard work and, if truth be told, it is often far harder work in Elinor's compassionate and accepting bubble than in the mute, awkward or combative sessions of my past.

I think it might be helpful to spend some time delving a little deeper into a few of the ways I have found therapy hard work even when I've been enjoying the process overall.

THE IMBALANCE OF POWER

Therapy can often feel uncomfortable due to the one-way aspect of the relationship. My therapist, for example, knows more about me than the vast majority of my friends do and she arguably knows me even better than I know myself at times, but it is not reciprocal. She doesn't share her worries, vulnerabilities and problems with me and I know very little about her, whereas I share so much of my personal life with her. This can make you feel really weird and a bit off-balance at times.

I have to admit that I find myself spending a fair proportion of the time holding back questions about her. Not just what big stuff might be going on in her life and what she's juggling, but I find my mind wandering on to the boring little stuff like what she does in her spare time, what inside her house looks like, what foods she likes, whether she travels, what drew her to therapy, and what she talks to her own therapist about.

Every therapist will vary on the amount of personal information they share with their clients – some might prefer to be a total blank slate, while others might use their own experiences to connect with you. For example, they might open up about a shared experience in order to show you empathy, normalise your experiences or to suggest something that they think might help your situation that has worked for them.

The relatively one-way aspect of therapy does not mean only one of you is doing the work. Your therapist will also be working hard to keep clear boundaries so that they can emotionally hold a safe space for you to heal. Therapy is most definitely a team pursuit, but with your change, growth and challenges at the very core.

DIFFICULTIES WITH TRUST

So many of us have been taught, usually subconsciously, not to show vulnerability. Boys are often told from a young age to 'man up' while girls are told to 'not make a fuss'. We are conditioned by others, but also as a human survival and coping strategy, not to show weakness or vulnerability, but therapy is inherently, at its heart, a vulnerable activity. Therefore, it's completely understandable to feel uncomfortable in expressing our emotions honestly, particularly if we are new to showing such vulnerability to others and are worried that we're opening up a Pandora's box of pain that once out could do more harm than good. This also means that it can take us quite some time to open up and trust our therapist.

But trust is rarely an instantaneous part of any relationship. You might have initially good feelings about your therapist, but deep trust takes time to build. It is often a slow dance of revealing just a little bit of ourselves at a time and seeing how the therapist reacts. Do they meet our pain or disclosures with honesty, compassion and empathy? If they do, we then often feel confident enough to reveal a little bit more, and so on.

WEIRD WORRIES

Worries, in every imaginable flavour, thrum with an endless rat-tat-tat around and around my mind:

▶ I worry she will think I'm pathetic.

▶ I worry she will think I can't handle my life.

▶ I worry about how to choose what to talk about.

▶ I worry she is going to judge me for what I bring up.

▶ I worry that I won't use the time effectively, and that I'll come out of each session feeling like I've spent £50 on something unnecessary.

EVEN MORE SECRET WORRIES

▶ What if I bore her?

▶ What if she hates me?

▶ What if she laughs at me?

▶ What if she thinks I'm crazy?

▶ What if she thinks I'm not crazy enough?

▶ What if I am wasting my time and my money?

▶ What if she is wasting my time and my money?

▶ What if I am beyond help?

GETTING STUCK

My main worry is that I won't know what to say. Even now, years into having therapy weekly, I still feel the familiar prickles of apprehension before the start of each session about what exactly will unfold. What will happen if I draw a blank? What if I miss something critical that is the key to unlocking the messy chaos of my mind? What if I fail to articulate the feeling properly? Which of my thoughts are more important – am I wasting my time bringing up my stressful meeting when I should be talking about my childhood? Even when things are going well and the conversation is flowing, the fear is constantly niggling away in the background: what happens if this river of insight suddenly dries up and I'm left staring at the wall unable to find the right words?

And it's not theoretical, it does actually happen. Usually after a particularly triumphant session where I've discovered all sorts of things about myself and perhaps even experienced a rare light bulb of insight, when the next session rolls around, I find I often draw a complete blank on where to start. The easy breezy flow of the previous week has vanished, replaced with awkward silence. None of the topics we've covered before seem very interesting or important, and nothing new comes to mind. I ask myself if maybe therapy isn't working, or if I've done all I can and maybe now it's time to stop. I even worry about disappointing Elinor; that, heaven forbid, she will start to see me as a difficult client. I do *not* want to be a difficult client.

While these thoughts race through my head, I become even more aware of the ticking clock and the increasingly awkward silence in the room. Part of me wants the session to end mercifully soon, while another part wants to figure this out and get back to the good work we were doing the previous week.

That's not to say that silence during therapy is always a bad thing. Sure, it can be unnerving when you don't know what to say and the searing light of the third degree makes you feel like a deer caught in the headlights, but in more recent times there have been moments when I have found the silences during therapy to be useful or, dare I say it, even comforting. Silence can be golden.

- I am a people-pleaser with a strong need to perform and achieve, which can and does extend into wanting to dazzle my therapist with an intriguing problem, fascinating insight or dramatic story. So to actually sit and do nothing for a few minutes, allowing the silence to hang in the air between us without me rushing to instantly fill it, has been excruciating but also some of the most enriching work I have done in therapy.

- Although it can feel awkward sometimes, it's enough just to feel the emotion without speaking. There's something rather lovely, for me anyway, about not always hurrying to put into words my feelings, especially when those feelings are heavy or tricky in some way.

- Therapy does provide moments of real clarity or insight – the mic drop, the truth bomb, the 'aha' moment, the penny drop, the light bulb of realisation – that sometimes need a few moments to digest.

JO'S TOOLKIT: MY TIPS ON BECOMING UNSTUCK

▶ *Talk it out.* Rather than silently getting more and more stuck on the feeling of being stuck, I've found it helpful to voice out loud that I'm feeling stuck. Often just addressing the feeling of not knowing what to say throws up some insights as to why I might be feeling blocked. Am I protecting or sabotaging myself somehow? Why is it I feel stuck today? Has something happened? Or maybe there is something I'm not ready to talk about yet. Why is that?

▶ *Be an early bird.* It doesn't always work out this way of course, but I do try to get to my appointment a little bit ahead of time to help clear my thoughts and think about what I might want to discuss. It's sometimes really hard to downshift into therapy mode when I'm in a rush, have battled rush-hour traffic, couldn't find a parking space or I am generally in a flap about running late.

▶ *Make a note.* 'I had something I wanted to talk about today, but now I can't for the life of me remember what it was' is one of my most said and thought phrases in therapy. A new tactic I have is to jot it down as I think of it during the week.

▶ *Back to basics.* I have found that asking myself 'What do I want right now?' and 'How do I feel right now?' always wriggle me free of the stuckness.

▶ Remember it's OK, if you are truly stuck, to ask the therapist for help. But don't be too surprised if that help comes in the form of questions about why you are stuck rather than them throwing you a lifeline of chit-chat.

MY THERAPIST NOT TELLING ME WHAT TO DO

I have a fantasy of a session where I chat for a bit, ask my therapist what she thinks, she then tells me what to do, I go away and do it and it is as simple as that – I am fixed or the problem is solved. But of course, this has never happened and I'm not going to lie; at times, this is incredibly annoying. Questions about whether I should do this or that, go for that job or break up with that person, are often left unanswered, countered with further questions back from her. It's taken me a long time for the penny to drop that my therapist's job isn't about telling me exactly what to do, instead it is about encouraging me to find my own solutions.

MY THERAPIST TELLING ME WHAT TO DO

We may ask, we may beg, but if our therapists do end up telling us what to do, I've found the relief of having an answer quickly turns to resentment. My CBT days showed me this, when even the gentlest of guidance and smallest of suggestions felt enormously challenging and patronising. I think this is because ultimately as humans we want to have agency over our own lives, which is why as children we spend our time begging to make our own decisions rather than have them made for us.

Therapists may not give us advice, but they do give us guidance. They are trained to understand people and as such can help us sort out what we want to do, but they can't make our life choices for us. So, if there's one thing that we should also remember if we find ourselves frustrated by their advice or lack of, it is that the most powerful of truths, the ones we take the most seriously, are those we come to on our own.

JO'S TOOLKIT: THREE THINGS TO REMEMBER WHEN THERAPY GETS HARD

1   *You have not failed.* It's perfectly normal for therapy to feel hard. I know it can be frustrating when you want to move forward, but progress in therapy is rarely linear, and setbacks or hard sessions don't negate your progress forward; in fact often they can help it more than you know.

2   *Slow progress is still progress.* You wouldn't expect to run a marathon at full speed with no breaks, right? Therapy often resembles a marathon more than a sprint.

3   *Listen to your gut.* If you feel overwhelmed or fried from the hard work of therapy, talk about it with your therapist. You might need to change things up or build a game plan together to find a pace that works for you. But if you still find yourself dreading your next session or feel like you've been pushed too far into a dark place, it might mean your therapist or this type of therapy isn't right for you, right now.

Sometimes working through a difficult emotion, entrenched belief or profound life experience feels like being stuck or like therapy isn't working. But when you're doing the hard work of healing deep-seated pain, those wounds don't necessarily heal in one fell swoop. Deeply held memories, feelings and beliefs tend to shape many aspects of our lives, and it often takes more than one session, maybe even months of sessions (or more), to fully rewire them, heal them and move on from them.

I'm not sure how much truth there is to the phrase 'It's always darkest just before the dawn', but I know that pain is part of the healing process. Therefore, in order to heal a wounded part of ourselves, having it witnessed, understood, given a voice and offered the opportunity can release its burden. Pain is an unavoidable, intrinsic part of the work in therapy, but on the other side of it can be amazing transformation. Hang in there. It really is worth the journey.

Therapy thoughts

Elinor tells me, '*Therapy is really hard work. It is like getting in a boxing ring with a heavyweight champion. I am always in awe of the courage that clients show in sessions. I think the magic comes in when clients can find compassion for themselves, when they realise that they are good enough.*'

Chapter Seven
THERAPY IS
Learning

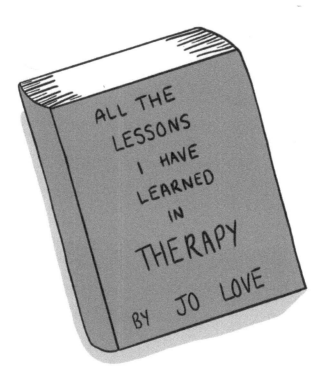

A huge misconception I held about therapy for many years, and I suspect I'm not alone on this one, is that therapists merely act as passive and, if I'm totally honest, expensive mirrors who don't actually say or do anything helpful or constructive, with empty utterances of 'Hmm, well how do *you* think you should feel?', 'Hmm, well what do *you* think you should have said?', 'Hmm, well how do *you* think your parents affected the way you view relationships?'

There will, of course, I'm sure, be people who do benefit hugely from this approach. However, I can confirm that I am not one of them. Yes, I need someone who listens to me and gives me space to heal, but I also need my therapy to be dynamic and collaborative. I need to learn and grow, and not just fill the air with my noise. No, for me, therapy must be active and constructive, with a pinch of self-disclosure on their part.

Therapy is all about learning. I've learned so many things over the years in the therapy room, from the tiny to the monumental, the blindingly obvious to the seemingly insignificant. As I've tunnelled inwards, I've blossomed outwards. Therapy has helped me grow awareness, understanding, responsibility and acceptance. It doesn't always make me feel better in the short term, but in the long term it does, helping me know who I am, why I do what I do and feel how I feel.

Before I deep dive into some of the bigger lessons I've learned, I'll kick off with a list of some of the smaller, but still hugely important, things my therapist has taught me:

- If you want to cry in your car, cry in your car.

- Sleep heals a hell of a lot.

- If you're panicking, breathe.

- If you're anxious, move.

- The word 'should' is not your friend.

- You're only responsible for your own shit, not anyone else's (tiny humans excluded).

- Most people find making, keeping and having friends hard.

- We all need coping mechanisms; the trick is to pick the healthy ones (therapy, self-care, meditation, nature, etc.) not the unhealthy ones (drugs, violence, denial, etc.).

- Being a human is hard, like really hard.

- The repair is always more important than the rupture.

Now for some of the big stuff I've learned in therapy...

DON'T FEAR THE FEELINGS

It seems a little silly to say this, but I didn't know before I was told explicitly in therapy that all emotions and feelings are OK. Yep, every single one. Even the ones I think of as 'bad' feelings or ones I shouldn't have. So that means even anger, fear, disgust, irritation, jealousy, sadness, anxiety... I could go on.

I remember the moment I learned this as clearly as if it were yesterday.

I am talking to Elinor about my brother returning to England after a few years living abroad with his wife and family. I had thought I was happy for his return, looking forward to seeing more of him and building new bonds with his growing family. But as I speak it dawns on me that I can feel visceral spikes of envy as we discuss how, on his return, he will be living far closer to my mum than I am presently. I explain to Elinor how I felt parallels with the story of the prodigal son when I heard the excited tone in my mum's voice when we spoke about his imminent return.

This feels so silly, so dramatic, and I am somewhat taken aback by my feelings of jealousy at my brother and, of course, what isn't, but what somehow feels very much like, a form of rejection from my mum. How can I be feeling this way? My head spins with confusion. I'm long past days of such petty sibling rivalry; after all, we are both grown adults with families of our own for goodness sake. This is something that surely I should have left far behind me in our childhoods. How petty of me to be jealous. How bitter and nasty I must be underneath it all to be feeling this way.

'I shouldn't be having these feelings; I should be able to cope. Other people would be able to deal with it far better than me,' I say with tear-soaked eyes.

When I stop my spiral of self-pity, Elinor says something that turns my world view upside down: 'You know, that sounds really quite normal.'

She tells me about her reversion into childish behaviours with her own brother each Christmas. It is comforting to hear this woman, who I respect and consider as having her shit together, tell me that she has experienced similar feelings, and clearly, on occasions, also doesn't quite have her shit together.

'Not only that,' she carries on, 'jealousy is completely and utterly OK.' She tells me that I needn't feel bad or guilty about it. I don't need to feel like I should be a bigger person. It is 'understandable'.

UNDERSTANDABLE.

This is a revelation.

'There are no negative or positive feelings,' she continues. 'Yes, sometimes there are feelings that hurt. Yes, they are hard;

yes, they are uncomfortable and can be difficult or tricky to manage at times, meaning we often label them as bad. But really, they are neither good nor bad. It's not about "should" and "should not" when it comes to emotions, they are all there to show us something. Usually something really rather helpful. Feeling them and noticing them is helpful. Pushing them away, or feeling like we shouldn't have them, is not.'

The penny drops.

The aha moment happens.

The light bulb switch is flicked.

Oh, I am *meant* to feel these things, all of them.

I had thought pain was for hiding, deflecting, ignoring, numbing, pushing down and away. I thought feelings were hard because I had done something wrong. I saw painful emotions as a weakness, a weakness I shouldn't have. A weakness that made me flawed, bad, wrong and not worthy.

Suddenly all those Pinterest platitudes make sense; it really is 'OK to feel *all* the feels'.

And do you know what? It really is.

Therapy has really helped me work on being brave enough to sit in the discomfort these emotions bring and really get curious about them until they have passed. Keeping the thoughts and feelings from my door has without a doubt provided me with a useful protection, but it is exhausting constantly keeping them at bay. Therapy has allowed me to gently, and with support, open the door, welcome them in, offer them a seat at my table, and in doing so I've seen they actually aren't all that big or that scary, and neither do they seem to hang around all that long, after all. Emotions move, emotions have motion. True, they might feel overwhelming for a while, but then they pass. They do pass.

Therapy has taught me how to not judge myself and feel guilty about having those feelings. Feeling bad about feeling bad.

Or meta emotions. A tiny example of this happened to me the other day.

I am running late and hop into my car only to find it won't start. Why won't the stupid car start, it's never done this before, why today? Then once it finally does start, this mood carries on. Why does every single traffic light seem to turn to red for me? Why am I stuck behind every slow driver on the road? Why does the world have it in for me?!

Then, I get mad at myself for getting mad. Why am I letting this ruin my day? Don't I know better by now? What's the point in doing all those meditations and breathing exercises if I go nuclear at the sight of a learner driver? I should be a bigger person. I should practise what I preach. I should be able to deal with this situation better. The guilt about not being patient, wasting my energy, not being who I expect me to be, and all the 'shoulds' floods over me.

Many of the things we all struggle with as human beings, while they feel like unique and inherent flaws to us, are in fact fairly universal. I really do believe that therapists are probably very uniquely placed to see all the unembellished truth of human nature, which gives them a truly accurate broad grasp of what it means to be normal. I trust Elinor when she says I'm normal.

And what I suspect the therapists would tell us if we asked is that normal is actually very far away from what we all insist on pretending it is.

★★★ JO'S TOOLKIT: A TINY TIP FOR BANISHING THE GUILT

A micro tip my therapist taught me for when I get the guilts about feeling a 'difficult' emotion is to put 'and that's OK' at the end of a tricky feeling or negative statement:

▶ 'I was annoyed at myself that I was running late... and that's OK.'

▶ 'I was angry the car wouldn't start... and that's OK.'

▶ 'I was frustrated all the traffic lights were red and the slow drivers were in my way... and that's OK.'

Or, doing it in the moment, which is more of a challenge, but super effective when I can manage it: 'I'm feeling a bit sad/ jealous/rejected/hurt/lost/alone right now... and that's OK.'

I AM LEARNING WHO I AM

I touched on this earlier, but I am unquestionably a serial people-pleaser. I am chronically helpful. I pride myself on being the capable one, the dependable one, the thoughtful one, the efficient one. And while it is, of course, a very normal human attribute to want to be liked by and connected to those around us, to shift ourselves slightly around different people we know in order to be accepted, I take this too far. I attend to the whims of others before my own, often leading me to take on more and more and not even notice when I've crossed the line into self-neglect and exhaustion.

It is still very much a work in progress for me, but therapy is helping me not only to learn where this has come from but also to unpick who I am underneath all the chameleon-like contortions I twist myself into.

From the Other Chair
PEOPLE-PLEASING

As Anna Mathur, psychotherapist (aka @annamathur on Instagram) and author of *Know Your Worth*, explains, people-pleasing isn't a mental illness in itself, but its influence on your life and relationships can be life-impacting. It's a challenging but worthy habit to tackle. Often the desire to make others happy has its roots in a deeper issue. For many, the eagerness to please stems from issues with their own self-worth. They hope that by saying yes to everything asked of them, they will feel worthy and liked. Other times, people-pleasers have a history of harm, mistreatment or abuse, and their way to survive was to please the people who mistreated them. Over time, this protective mechanism of people-pleasing has become the only way they know.

♥ JO'S TOOLKIT: SIGNS YOU MIGHT BE A PEOPLE-PLEASER

▶ You struggle to say 'no'.

▶ You find it hard to voice your opinion.

▶ You're always on the lookout for rejection.

▶ You often suffer at the expense of doing a favour for others.

▶ You feel like you are wearing a mask a lot of the time.

▶ You often act based on what 'other people think' of you.

▶ You struggle with your boundaries.

▶ You have low self-worth.

▶ You are empathetic to others, but rarely to yourself.

▶ You fear losing control.

Growing up, it felt like my parents, and my father in particular, prized my academic achievement above all else. What was said was, 'We want you to do more with your lives than we did with ours', but what therapy has helped me to see is that my small child brain heard that my father's love was tied to my performance academically.

He never said 'I will only love you if you succeed', but that message was reinforced many times over in subtle ways, so this is what I heard. I recall, aged seven, a teacher said I was average at maths; my father's reaction was that this was unacceptable on my part. I heard the disappointment, saw the displeasure; I felt the rejection and internalised it as shame. But then I would also see the pride, the happiness, the joy when I was excelling, when I became a straight-A student. I felt I had no choice than to keep this up.

What drove me to achieve wasn't a deep love for, or interest in every subject, but a desire to win the heart of a father who I felt was unable to tell the difference between loving me and loving my achievements, from separating the girl from the grades.

He would have no idea how much pressure he put on me to succeed. It would break his heart to know that I grew up believing his love for me was unconsciously conditioned on me excelling at everything I did and how scared I was of disappointing him, which then permeated into every aspect of my life. I pushed myself, perfection was the goal. I was hard on myself, probably far harder than he had ever been on me, and I never felt I could measure up. I never felt good enough. After all, living in a constant state of perfection is not possible to achieve.

Therapy has helped me to revisit and reshape these experiences. It's helped me to go back and speak directly to that seven-year-old girl and tell her a kinder, softer message. Tell her how her best was good enough, how she was loved no matter what she achieved. How she was absolutely wonderful just as she was.

The ripple effect of these experiences throughout my life has been examined and re-examined in the therapy room. Relearning what success actually is to me. Relearning who I am underneath the achievements, underneath all the masks.

'You must have loved your parents so very much to have left your true self behind to please them.'

She does it again.

BOOM, MIC DROP. PENNY DROP. AHA. LIGHT BULB. DING DING DING.

Love lies behind it all. I am not a bad person – there is not emptiness behind the masks. Far from emptiness in fact, there is love. Love was the reason, love is behind it all.

Slowly, piece by piece, one tiny step at a time, therapy is helping me begin to learn I am not the four lies I have been telling myself my whole life:

1   I am not what I do.

2   I am not what I have.

3   I am not what I achieve.

4   I am not what other people think about me.

One day I will be free of these lies.

Therapists have a way of dropping some seriously wise shit on you, some of which can stick with you for a long time. Some of the important lessons I've learned include:

▶ It's OK to fail. It's OK to mess up and make mistakes.

▶ Crying isn't giving up or a weakness, crying helps.

▶ Everything is temporary.

▶ The only person you can change is you. But by you changing, other people and things around you may well shift too.

▶ Most of the things you think of as my fault are not your fault.

▶ Healing and growth does not happen overnight and there is no finishing line.

▶ Happiness is in the now, or nowhere at all.

Therapy definitely isn't supposed to eradicate all sadness, anger, frustration or other negative emotions from our lives. And what I've learned is it's a good thing it doesn't, because often it's those tougher emotions that serve as important internal cues for us all. For me, that's part of the magic of therapy. Therapy is there to gently help me learn how to sit with, accept and not be debilitated by these feelings, all while cultivating self-awareness. The result? I've learned how to tune in and make choices that make the most sense for me.

Rather than achieving perpetual bliss, therapy is about learning how to more confidently be able to navigate life off the proverbial couch.

Therapy thoughts

Natasha Devon MBE, mental health and body image campaigner and writer, tells me that the biggest lesson she's learned from therapy is that 'not everything in life gets resolved and you have to learn to live with that or you'll go actually wall-climbing crackers'.

Chapter Eight
THERAPY IS
Magic

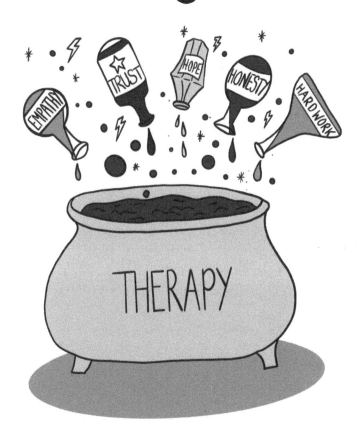

At this point in the book, I'm sure it will be abundantly clear to you that therapy is not a magical quick fix. Sadly, there is no wand that can be waved, no incantation to chant and no potion to drink so that all our problems will disappear in a puff of smoke.

Therapy is often hard. Therapy is often slow. Therapy can be painful. Therapy is frequently uncomfortable. But for me, what happens in therapy really does *feel like magic*.

The seemingly simple ingredients of one small room, two relative strangers, 50 minutes of time and some words spoken, has the power to raise my levels of emotional well-being, self-understanding, self-compassion and fulfilment, and dispels feelings of being lost, sad, angry, self-defeating and unconfident.

But how does it do this? Really, how?

In trying to answer this question, it might be helpful if I delve a little deeper and look at what makes therapy feel like pure magic for me.

I CAN TAKE OFF MY MASK

In Japan they have a proverb that we all have three faces: one we show to the world, one we show to our close friends and family, and another we never show to anyone. It is this last face that is the truest reflection of who we really are. For me, this certainly rings true: most of who we are is often kept secret from the world.

No one, no matter how close a relative, friend or lover, can ever really know more than a fraction of our inner workings. Sure, they can know parts of us or versions of ourselves pretty well, but it will only ever be a small part of who we actually are underneath it all. We gradually learn throughout our childhoods and upbringings to create protected boundaries between what we say out loud and what is truthfully going on inside our minds. We learn to mask much of our inner selves. And these masks shield us well.

For me, they work a little too well.

Without being aware that I am doing it, the masks have multiplied and mutated and often present only an illusion of myself to the world. An echo of what really lies within. One that I think fits best with other people's expectations of me. Masks that can flip, twist and change in a moment depending on who I am with, what I am doing and where I am. On the outside I show everyone how 'together' I am and how life isn't fazing me at all. Meanwhile, on the inside, the real me is silently screaming out for help as I spin out of control.

My most-used masks include:

▶ The 'I'm OK' mask, often used when the reality is that I am feeling anything but OK.

▶ The 'I'm bright and bubbly' mask, which I find to be particularly useful when I'm feeling lonely and depressed.

▶ The 'I'm here for you' mask, when what I really need is for someone to be there for me.

▶ The 'I'm calm, confident and in control' mask, regularly deployed when I'm feeling anxious and out of control.

These masks aren't about trying to deceive people. For me they are more about protection and self-preservation. Without conscious thought or planning I am pulling on the layers to cover up myself from the world. From the hurt.

And gosh it's exhausting. It's almost impossible to describe just how much energy and effort goes into every interaction in order to make other people more comfortable with me. The toll it takes is enormous.

But in therapy the masks can come off. I can say what I want, and a good therapist will actively encourage it. Inside the safety of the therapy room, I have found I can let my true skin breathe and tell someone what I really feel like inside, no matter how odd, frightening or dark.

The vulnerability this requires can be quite a challenge, especially if you're not used to it, but by someone to listening to us, not judging us, encouraging and supporting us, believing in us and sticking with us, the whole process can be a less daunting one.

Remember, there's no need to throw away the masks straight away. They can come off slowly and only when you are ready and feel safe enough to do so. Be kind to yourself and take it one step at a time.

I CAN TALK ABOUT WHAT I WANT TO

Sometimes I will want to deep dive, dig around in my past, my childhood, my parents, my friends, my traumas. Forensically examine the unique set of patterns and behaviours that make me, me. Try to place where they all come from, connect the dots, piece together the jigsaw pieces of my life in order to grab on to who I am that little bit tighter. Sometimes I will want to rant and rave about politics and the state of the world or find myself in existential crisis about who I am, how I fit into the world and what my life purpose is. Other times I will lament about my husband not picking up his socks or how I completely lost my shit in that group WhatsApp chat.

This is all part of the magic for me. Therapy is exactly what I want it to be. No topic is too big, no topic is off limits, nothing is too stupid, too small or too trivial. It's all permitted – the inner workings of your mind in all their messy, glorious detail for another to see.

I HAVE MY OWN TEAM

One of the truly great feelings I get from therapy is having my very own 'Team Jo'. My therapist is on my side in a way that is both comforting and refreshingly consistent. She is someone who brings me a focused and generous attention week after week, in a way that we so rarely experience outside of the therapy room. Even our closest and most loyal friends, family or lovers will find themselves at times to be bored, distracted, envious or keen to project their own views or values on to our lives.

But in the therapy room it is different. We talk about what I want to talk about. She sees my life through my eyes. She is sorry if I have suffered, she understands if something was scary, or worrying, or stressful, or upsetting. I have found that knowing I have someone in my corner allows me to think and speak, without being influenced by other people's thoughts, feelings or actions. It gives me the much-needed freedom to get some clarity on my true feelings and thoughts and have the courage to face the vulnerabilities that I'd otherwise prefer to bury or build defences against.

This is not to say she agrees with everything I say. Far from it, in fact. But the difference is, even when I am challenged by her, it is done with empathy, kindness and care, meaning I don't feel judged, shamed or defensive. It feels safe. It is not combative. And because it feels so safe, it opens the door for new possibilities and allows the space for how I really feel about things to emerge.

I CAN CONNECT THE DOTS

When left to my own devices my brain is prone to meandering. I often get lost and lose my train of thought, or find myself going round and round in metaphorical circles, or become too closely knotted up in the heat of the emotion. Irrelevant ideas have a habit of flitting in and out of my mind, often scrambling my tentative insights.

But in therapy, the spotlight of my therapist's focus gives me the confidence to remain curious about the more slippery concepts, however peculiar or out of reach from me they may feel. The very lightest of pressure from the outside to remain focused on the thought, intriguingly and somewhat magically, seems to straighten some of the tangled ideas within. I still stumble, repeat things and get confused, but she's there guiding me gently back to the ground I missed, sidestepped or rushed over.

She is the keeper of all the threads, she keeps me on track and connects the dots. She unearths the roots of the tree (my past) and connects them to the branches and leaves of the stories I present to her, leaf by leaf, branch by branch.

I HAVE A WITNESS

In telling my therapist my story, I can see the reaction of someone else to my pain, my dark parts, my shame. The things I usually keep carefully hidden away from the world are now public. Sure, not public public, I haven't stood on a podium and told the world my most secret thoughts, but they are public in the sense that they have left my private inner world where they like to metastasise and stagnate, and are now in the safe air of the therapy room. They now have a witness. A witness who, if the therapist is doing their job right, isn't horrified into running for the hills by these confessions, but instead reacts with a calm, supportive interest. I am no longer carrying them alone, I am unburdened. I am lighter somehow.

And now there is a new version of my story, one that includes this safe external witness. And I can see it from her perspective where it looks smaller, less scary, more benign somehow. Crucially, I learn I am not a monster or a freak. I learn I am not alone or a reject. I am less opaque to myself. Less fragile. She is there with me.

I CAN QUIETEN MY INNER CRITIC

Inside of me lives a Shirley (sorry to any Shirleys who might be reading this book). Shirley is the name I give to this constant, negative, nagging little inner voice. So named because of a childhood neighbour, Shirley, who exhibited many of the qualities I have attributed to my internal 'Shirley'. You know the type – a spiteful, toxic, judgemental, complaining sort of person. Someone who is always sticking their nose into your business, perpetually on the hunt for things you have done wrong, watching and waiting for you to take a misstep so they can then gleefully swoop in and, in the most public way possible, admonish you for your crime. She's always there, Shirley, surveilling what I do, studying how I perform, examining how I interact with others, tracking my successes and failures. She's not the silent type either. Oh no, she's a 'demand to speak to the manager' type person. She loudly booms her critical verdicts of damnation about how I should have done this or that better, all with a tone of deep contempt that I cannot ignore.

She is punitive, she is humiliating.

Shirley is a bitch.

Therapy provides me with an alternative, softer, kinder perspective and new information, which often disrupts Shirley in her tracks. My therapist identifies when I am being critical of myself in ways that aren't fair and offers a counter-narrative to the negative thoughts.

I have found that I can now 'catch Shirley in the act' and identify when I am being unfair in my self-reflection. And without really realising it, I have started to slowly shift the dialogue. So now instead of listening to Shirley when something doesn't go to plan or I feel I could have done something better, I've heard myself saying, 'What would my therapist say?' having heard her constructive, kindly voice so often tackling such a range of tricky issues.

Shirley, who had once manifested as unconquerable and unkind, has begun to shrink and shrivel. Her power has lifted, her dominance diminished.

I HAVE LIGHT-BULB MOMENTS

No list of why therapy feels like magic could be complete without mentioning the 'light-bulb' moments, the 'aha' moments, the 'penny drop' moments, the 'epiphanies'. Those times the little hairs on your arms stand up or when something clicks and you look at life in a different way to how you did only moments before. Whatever you want to call them, these moments are often thought of as the Holy Grail of therapy, but they are often sorely misunderstood.

Six realisations I've had about therapy light bulbs:

1   They are nowhere near as frequent as the movies and TV shows would have you believe.

2   You think you've never thought of it that way before, but you can't have a light bulb unless you already knew it deep down somewhere. The light bulb is the awakening, the remembering, the awareness of what you already knew, articulated in a way that resonates with your own truth.

3   Light-bulb moments are not the destination for therapy; they are less the finishing line and more akin to the first day of training for a triathlon. Because just as you identify a pattern, a reason for behaving a certain way or a change you want to make, it often means the real therapeutic work towards a larger goal is just beginning.

4   There's no magical number of hours you need spend on the couch, correct words you can say or step-by-step formula you need follow that will lead you to having one of these light-bulb moments.

5   Some people will never have a one-off light-bulb moment; instead they experience a more subtle slow creep of change in their lives as a result of therapy.

6   You get to decide what a breakthrough looks or feels like to you. I've tried to explain my light bulbs to other people in the past and they always sound so obvious when I say them out loud. I have found it almost impossible to articulate the seismic power they have held and their ability to rock my core views.

I MAKE SLOW AND STEADY PROGRESS

Perhaps more magical than the elusive light-bulb moments is actually a slow, steady, incremental, transformational crawl towards change. Although I don't disagree that short-term therapy can be enormously beneficial for some people and for some issues, for me I have come to appreciate the slower pace of decoding myself over the longer term. Personally, I've never felt able to fully convey my key experiences in only a few self-contained blocks of time; some weeks I'm tightly wound and unable to create much slack in the wire, whereas others I feel readier to unravel certain memories or consider other viewpoints. While at times it can be frustrating not to be constantly making leaps and bounds forward, I have come to enjoy the slower, carefully considered pace of piecing together the unearthed fragments from the mounds of debris.

I FIND THE WORDS

Somehow being forced to articulate my feelings and experiences to another person often allows me to grasp them in a clearer way. Very often my sessions are the process of working out whether the words that have emerged are the right ones. I often say things like, 'No, that's not quite right.' They often need swapping, refining, rejigging. Sometimes the words that come out are comforting, but also they can be unexpected and, at times, alarming.

It can be shocking and confronting when some of the words and feelings are eventually said aloud; externalising what has previously been internal and hearing the private parts that live inside us reverberating around the therapy room. It's always been illuminating for me how tricky some topics are to articulate even as a seasoned therapy client. I find it usually arises when I have to say something nice about myself: 'Why am I squirming?' I squeak. 'Gosh, I really do find this so hard to say out loud, even in here.'

Talking about language, the words used by my therapist are

careful, considered and often packed with insight. She has an incredible way of asking a question, for example, and my answer may not be important, per se, but it is more about what it opens up for me, what it unlocks, what path it then sends me down. Though her actual words frustratingly slip and fade away from me as soon as I leave my session, I think they do exist within me on a subconscious level for when I need to draw on them. Or perhaps the words themselves are inconsequential but where those words take me is really where the magic lies.

SOME PRECIOUS GEMS GIVEN TO ME BY MY THERAPIST THAT I FREQUENTLY REMIND MYSELF OF WHEN TIMES GET TOUGH ARE:

▶ 'That must have been really hard for you.'

▶ 'It sounds like you're carrying a lot right now.'

▶ 'You are doing so well.'

▶ 'That is a lot to deal with.'

▶ 'So many other people also struggle with exactly this.'

▶ 'Be gentle with yourself.'

I HAVE A BOND

Last but most definitely not least is the bond between me and the therapist – the trust, the empathy, the way I feel seen, heard and understood.

That said, my therapist is not and can never be my friend. I will never meet her for a coffee, we will never watch TV together, go see a movie or do any number of other normal activities, but we do, without a shadow of a doubt, have a relationship; a relationship that is more intimate than any other I've experienced in a professional service context. (With a quick aside, I do think it's worth mentioning how certain service providers, such as taxi drivers, hairdressers, personal trainers or beauticians, often find themselves in pseudo-therapist roles. While I have certainly felt echoes of the therapeutic relationship with some of these, they have never fully recreated that magical alchemy of therapy for me, mainly as their opinions and problems are never truly absent, like they so often are in therapy.)

For me, the unique alliance forged between the helper and the helped is where the magic really happens. It's the very essence of its power.

It is empathetic and genuine.
It is intimate and accepting.
It is unbiased and impartial.
It is transparent and non-judgemental.
It is protected and secure.
It is respectful and considerate.
It is unique and collaborative.

Over the years, research has consistently confirmed that the therapeutic relationship, or as some call it the therapeutic alliance, itself is essential to the success of therapy. Some studies have even called this therapeutic alliance the most important common factor in having a successful outcome in therapy.

From the Other Chair
THE THERAPEUTIC RELATIONSHIP AND TRANSFERENCE

As Dr Tina Mistry, clinical psychologist (aka @brownpsychologist on Instagram), explains, if your therapist has the capacity to really lean into what you are going through this helps, but also they need the ability to stay open to getting it wrong. Above all, as a therapist I have learned that staying humble and human is the key. I often say to clients, 'you are the expert on your life; I know some psychology stuff and our job is to bring that knowledge together'. The aim of this is to remove any power hierarchy dynamic, which can be present in the relationship. For me, there is power in curiosity and not knowing, and being open about that. It offers a space where we can be collaborative and equal, while showing our clients that we care and want them to grow.

Developing and maintaining a therapeutic relationship requires constant and consistent work. We have to check in with ourselves as therapists and with how we feel the relationship is with our clients. We need courage to ask our clients how they feel the relationship is going, making it explicit and sitting with the discomfort of working through any ruptures.

This is because the relationship is not only essential but can also be a focus of therapy itself. The way we treat our therapist can give them clues to our past as we replay our histories within our therapeutic relationship. This is known as 'transference'. It occurs when we project our feelings about someone else, someone we have encountered in our pasts, on to our therapist. It can sometimes be an obstacle in therapy, particularly if it becomes a barrier to getting help because you have fallen in love with your therapist or are very angry with or distrustful of them, for example. However, this is not always the case, as the way we interact with our therapist can often offer us a chance to experience a new and corrective relationship that actually heals some of these old wounds.

HOW THE MAGIC ACTUALLY HAPPENS

When writing this book, I started to get curious about how therapy actually works, how it goes about healing us, how it is that two people talking to each other actually creates change. I do sort of get it; it makes a certain amount of sense to me that opening up to a trained, non-judgemental listener, speaking the previously unspoken, has enormous healing benefits. But this is based on how I *feel* it works, and not how it *actually* works.

There is a large body of academic research showing that people who get help and support from therapy are generally emotionally better off than those who do not. But I still found myself needing to know what the mechanics are – why exactly does it make people feel better?

I needed an answer, and after many hours poring over the research, I managed to find one. It's not an easy answer mind you, so I'm going to split in into two parts.

THE MAGICAL INGREDIENTS

Researchers have identified four main ingredients, the presence of which can be used to estimate how well therapy will work on a person. These are:

1 *The 'you' factor.* According to the researchers, this accounts for roughly 40 per cent of change in therapy. Elements such as how we as clients engage in the process, how open we are, how much motivation we have and what we want to get out of therapy all impact how much it actually works. This is basically the idea that therapists don't change us, we change with the help of therapy.

2 *The 'relationship' factor.* The quality of the relationship between us as the client and our therapists accounts for approximately 30 per cent of what makes therapy work. Elements such as the level of empathy, warmth and encouragement received will help with how effective therapy is for us.

3 *The 'hope' factor.* This accounts for about 15 per cent. It's worth noting that this doesn't need to be a total blind faith in the process as it's normal to be slightly sceptical about therapy, but a hope that therapy might make a positive difference will itself have an impact.

4 *The 'technique' factor.* The therapist's technique accounts for the remaining 15 per cent. As we will explore in more detail in Chapter Ten, there are many different techniques and types of therapy. And there is evidence that certain techniques are more helpful for certain issues, but what is more important than the technique is

that your therapist's way of helping feels comfortable and makes sense to you.

HOW NEUROSCIENCE GETS INVOLVED

The second part of the answer lies in the complex and still-emerging world of neuroscience and neurobiology – looking at how therapy works to alter our brains.

It's at this point that I should probably admit to you that this is where I slipped down a metaphorical neuroscience-shaped rabbit hole that I found quite tricky to navigate my way out of. I was equally fascinated and bamboozled. Every new book, article and piece of research I read led me to another book, article and piece of research, of which I understood very little. Intellectually curious as I am, neuroscientist I am not, but I felt duty-bound to plough on. It was actually my own therapist who managed to rescue me as I increasingly tied myself in neurobiological knots. She helped me realise that it is not my job, nor the job of this book, to explain neuroscience, or indeed therapy, to you, but what I can do is tell you my experiences and what I've taken away from this geeky rabbit hole adventure. With that in mind, here goes with a hugely oversimplified explanation of what I gleaned:

From day one, humans are born vulnerable and we must depend on others to survive. We are born unable to walk, speak or perform many cognitive tasks. As such, our brains have evolved to mean we are born equipped and ready to engage in relationships, even if it is only through crying out for our caregivers. Our brains therefore are inescapably social from their first moments in the world, and their structure and function are deeply embedded within groups of other brains, i.e. our parents, families, tribes and societies.

And this, in its simplest form, is what is at the heart of the link between psychotherapy and neurobiology. The ability of the therapist to connect with and attune to us will actually help build new neural connections in the brains of us, their clients, helping us to adapt and change.

What's very cool about therapy is the potential for it to change our brains on a structural level. The brain and nerve circuitry are much more malleable, or plastic, than previously supposed, where the thought was once we reached a certain age that was us, and our brains, set in our ways for life. But it turns out that rewiring is very much possible in adult life. Maybe not always easy (ever heard the phrase 'You can't teach an old dog new tricks'?), but we do know now that it is possible.

This change in the functional architecture of our brains, creating new neurons or pathways, is called 'neuroplasticity'. Although neuroplasticity hasn't been understood until relatively recently, it has actually been very much in action in the therapy room for hundreds of years, with therapists using their connection and skill in order to galvanise change in their clients, well before it was ever discovered what they were in fact doing on a neurobiological level.

When we spend time in therapy, talking in a way that is open, safe and attuned, our brain and our subconscious get slowly cajoled into new thoughts, reactions and awareness. So, where we might have formed ideas that feel fixed, such as 'this will always be the way', 'things will never change' or my favourite 'this is just who I am', as our subconscious gets more airtime, we have the option to release long-held ideas that may not benefit our own well-being. What happens, in a very subtle way, is the opening of new neural pathways, which in turn changes our brain's architecture.

Another way in which therapists can change our brains is by modelling how to respond to situations or thought patterns in a more positive way than we are currently attempting. The very act of observing a therapist approach a problem in a different, positive way can and does activate something called mirror neurons. The activation of these mirror neurons on repeated occasions actually strengthens the pathways in our own brains, meaning next time we are presented with the same issue or problem we won't take the old path but will mirror the more positive route we have learned. Much like going to the gym and building our muscles, the more we use these new pathways, the stronger they become and, crucially, the easier they are for us to use the next time we need them.

Boiled right down, the very process of telling our story, self-reflection and watching our therapist mirror positive reactions, can and does make small incremental structural changes in our brains and helps us change and grow.

Quite literally my tiny mind was blown!

But neuroscience cannot be the whole answer. Therapists will always be relying on their skill, intuition and experience in order to tune into and reveal the subtle and hidden conflicts and emotions that could never be revealed in even the most sophisticated of brain scans.

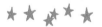

I'm not ashamed to admit that I have become really quite evangelical about the transformative effects of therapy. I feel compelled to lift the veil of secrecy and shame and let people into the revelation that therapy isn't all about mental illness, it's about growth. I wish more people knew how it is supposed to feel. My therapist is a bit like a physiotherapist for my mind, diligently and meticulously helping me to recover from an injury, week-by-week building and repairing damaged muscles, increasing my strength and providing me with the tools and guidance for my own self-healing and protection from future injury.

Therapy has changed my life because therapy is about life. All of my life. No problem or issue is too big or too small for the therapy room. Some weeks I get deep into heavy topics such as grief, death, PTSD or suicide, while others I chat about toxic friends, narcissistic bosses or my husband's inability to put his own clothes in the goddamn washing machine. And that is part of the magic of therapy that no one seems to be talking about but that has been hugely healing for me. Everything is connected, everything is important.

I wish I had known this earlier.

Therapy thoughts

'Therapy has transformed the way I think about myself, life events and given me the space to be totally honest. It has allowed me to accept so much more about myself, my recovery but also my relationships. Therapy is magic because it gives us the strength to keep fighting even when we feel like giving up.'
Hope Virgo, leading eating disorder campaigner and author

Part Two

GETTING THE MOST OUT OF THERAPY

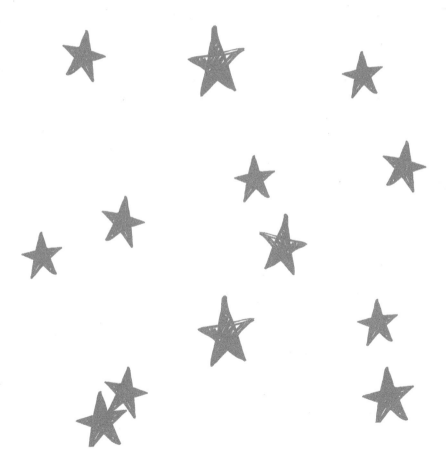

Chapter Nine
IS THERAPY
For You?

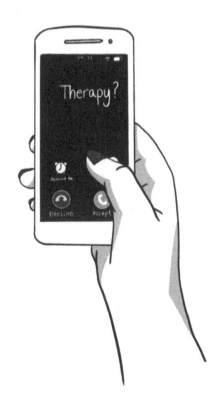

The next few chapters will explore how you can find and access therapy, what to expect and a little bit about what to look for, what questions you might want to ask and how to prepare for that nerve-racking first session. But before we dig into all that, you need to ask yourself whether therapy is really for you.

Not everyone needs therapy, and therapy won't always be the right course for all people at all stages of their lives, but I do believe that the vast majority of people can benefit from therapy, provided they are with the right therapist for them and receive the correct therapy (more on this below).

WHY GO TO THERAPY?

I truly believe therapy is always worth exploring as it can provide a safe place to delve into so many different issues and aspects of our lives, such as:

▶ Feeling stuck or unfulfilled.

▶ Feeling a bit sad, worn out, burned out, lost or just a bit 'meh'.

▶ Dealing with difficult or toxic friends, family or influences in your life.

▶ Dealing with changes and life transitions.

▶ You want a safe place to practise being more assertive, more social, more vulnerable, more *something*.

▶ You need help healing some old wounds or learning how to forgive.

▶ You want to improve your relationships to be a better friend, partner, child or parent.

▶ You are suffering with anxiety, depression, low self-esteem, unresolved grief or bullying.

▶ You want to become more self-aware and emotionally intelligent and learn new skills or strategies.

▶ For no reason at all, you just fancy trying it out.

No list such as this could ever be complete, and it's unusual to be in therapy for just one of these reasons – we often go to address several concerns. Some might say that broadly all of these could be put into two general categories: issues in our relationships with others and issues in our relationship with ourselves. Something that's often not talked about is seeking out therapy not for an issue, but for a more positive rationale, for example to give yourself a space to seek out joy or celebrate your successes.

Personally, I've often landed in therapy due to feeling like I've got something wrong or failed at something in my life, but what I have found is that therapy turns this way of thinking on its head.

I went to therapy expecting to get fixed, but what I have learned is that I was never broken.

WHEN IS THE RIGHT TIME?

As I've said many times in this book, it is my firm belief that therapy can help the vast majority of people, if it is the right time, the right therapy and the right therapist for that individual and what they need from therapy. In an ideal world, it's probably better to try to seek out therapy when you're not really struggling but rather when you first start to notice signs of something not being quite right or that there's something you'd like to explore. This is far easier said than done though, particularly if you are looking to receive therapy through the NHS. I've often felt that trying to look for therapy when you are in the depths of mental distress is a little like trying to locate the stopcock when your house has already flooded.

Therapy isn't just for moments of earth-shattering personal tragedy; it's not always for rock-bottom/crisis points. It can also be useful in reorienting yourself towards your true wants and needs, training yourself in the art of self-compassion, and better understanding, respecting and communicating your feelings. And guess what, it's often easier to reach these goals when you're not wrestling bigger, darker obstacles. So consider this

A very important side note on being in crisis: while therapy can help people work through issues that lead to thoughts of suicide, it's usually not the best option for people actually in crisis and actively wanting to end their lives. If you are in crisis, you can get help right away by reaching out to a suicide helpline through phone, text message or online chat. You may be encouraged to call or visit the nearest A&E. A therapist can help support you going forward, once you are no longer in crisis.

If you ever feel as though you are unable to keep yourself safe, you should immediately call 999 or go to your local A&E. This won't always mean you are sent to hospital, as most mental health trusts have something called Crisis or Home Treatment Teams, who can look after you by visiting you regularly in your own home and being on call 24 hours a day.

A full list of crisis resources is listed on page 260.

your permission to give therapy a try, even if you feel your life is going hunky-dory. Your future self may just look back and thank you for it.

HOW DO I KNOW I AM READY?

Entering therapy before you are ready is not something I'd advise; I've been there and got the T-shirt and smelled the stinky boots to boot. It's such a deeply personal and often challenging process, I found out the hard way that it really doesn't work unless you're ready.

Therapy is not something anyone takes on lightly – I've found that it always involves some degree of soul-searching and a considered thought process, which it goes without saying will be different for everyone. But how do you know if you are ready or not? The answer to this will be deeply personal, but two things I wish I had been asked, or asked myself prior to my disastrous therapy sessions before I was ready, would have been:

1. Am I looking for and am I open to change?
If the answer is 'No, I'm not', the timing might not be right for you at the moment. Perhaps you feel fine as you are and change isn't something you want to do right now, and that's OK. For therapy to be effective it does require an openness and a willingness to challenge one's thoughts, biases and preconceptions. So if you have been considering therapy and feel open to an honest dialogue with a therapist, you may find the process deeply rewarding.

2. Am I willing to be honest and vulnerable?
In order for therapy to benefit you, you will need to be able to

trust your therapist and open up. It might take some time to be able to do this, but it will be essential that you do. There have been times in my life when I haven't been ready to do this and that's OK.

That said, nerves are perfectly normal. Whether you've been to therapy before or this is the first time you're thinking about it, it can feel really unnatural at first to expose all your secrets and truths to a total stranger when perhaps you've previously dedicated so much energy to keeping everything bottled up inside. But I promise, the more you practise it, the easier it will become.

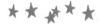

If you're thinking about therapy, take a moment to reflect and consider these questions. From my experience, when the time is right, you might be nervous and have questions and apprehensions, all of which are very normal, but you'll know.

Am I being forced into therapy?

Another thing to consider when asking yourself whether you are ready for therapy is whether you are doing it of your own free will.

It's safe to say that my grief counselling (and I think my counsellor would also agree with me on this) was a spectacular flop. This had almost nothing to do with her and her skills, but more to do with me and my reluctance to be there.

If you're forced into therapy for any reason – maybe loved ones are putting pressure on you or, like me, you find yourself having to attend in order to tick some bureaucratic box – it doesn't mean it's definitely going to fail, but it really doesn't set things off on the right foot. In my experience, it's only been when I have freely sought help and support from therapy that I have had the best outcomes.

EXCUSES FOR NOT GOING TO THERAPY

My therapy road has definitely been potholed with excuses, some legitimate and others less so. The research clearly shows that many people who very much need therapy often delay actively seeking treatment, usually by a factor of many years. Rather insidiously, many of our excuses often stem from the very same issues we need to seek help for. This might look like, *'I'm too depressed to get out of bed, let alone go to therapy'* or *'How could I trust someone enough to talk about my trust issues?'* Or maybe you need to talk to someone about your workplace anxiety, but you're too busy with work to make it to your therapy sessions.

Below is a list of crap excuses I've made for not going to therapy and exactly why they are crap:

I'm too tired
Hell yes, I'm tired. I am constantly tired. Not just sleepy tired – I'm a mum so that is par for the course. No, I'm tired of it all. I'm tired of scrolling and comparing, tired of an overwhelming news cycle, tired of giving myself a hard time for being so goddamn tired.

It can feel like I have a weight physically pummelling down on my shoulders and it's exhausting and there is nowhere to put it. But in the therapy room, I've found that talking it out takes some of the weighty energy out of some of my stress triggers and, rather remarkably, by doing so, the tired fog starts to lift.

I'm too busy
We live in a busy world; we are all busy, so busy. But I felt like I was the busiest, without a doubt. Therapy, pah! Wouldn't that be a lovely luxury?! But was I really *that* busy? I still managed to find plenty of time to binge-watch box sets, see my friends,

spend hours on Etsy looking at everything from pompom wicker baskets to rainbow dog leads, but leaving the house for therapy, that was too much. No, I wasn't too busy, maybe I was just not that interested in making time for therapy. Or was I too scared?

The fact of the matter is, we all have the same number of hours in a day, the same number of days in a week. Time is our currency to spend, and there is always time for things we believe are valuable enough to spend it on. Personally, I've found that with therapy, like many other things in life, the return on investment is huge. Call it self-care, call it maintenance, but if you think you don't have the time to spend on something that is going to benefit your entire life, that's something to think about.

I don't know how to find anyone

Even though I've used this excuse in the past – and I get it, it's confusing, it really is – I'm afraid you can't because you have this book and in it are all the answers.

It's for the crazy people, not me

Newsflash Jo. You might just be one of the crazy people! After all, we are all a little crazy underneath it all.

But seriously, this is an extremely common fear. So many of us think therapy is only for those who are really struggling or who we believe have been through something 'bad enough' to warrant it.

But here's the thing – the really bloody important thing that I wish I had known far earlier – all of our experiences are relative. They cannot be compared to anyone else's. We are the sum of our own experiences, no one else's. We all do it, but there is no use in measuring our difficulties against another person's. If we are feeling pain, we are feeling pain. If we are struggling and others might not be, or they are struggling more, that doesn't matter one jot, they are not us, we are still struggling and we still deserve help and support.

What will other people think?!

I hate, like really, really hate, admitting to anyone that I need help. I don't want to be someone who needs help. I want to be capable and competent. And if I do need help, I want to be able to help *myself* without having to alert ANYONE else to the fact that I might be struggling with something. Public admittance of a problem has for a very long time been an absolute no-go zone for me. It follows then that the very last thing I would want to do is tell someone else, 'Hey, I'm not coping – I think I need your help', which is essentially what going to therapy is.

But guess what, yes growth is deeply personal, but rarely ever is it solitary. We need to connect and share with others. When we do this something amazingly healing happens.

This doesn't stop me caring what other people think. Caring, probably far too much, about what other people think is one of the main reasons I ended up in therapy to begin with and why I am in therapy even to this day. But as uncomfortable as it is, people will make judgements – it's human nature for us all to appraise other humans. Meaning there will be some who accept therapy as a legitimate, normal and bold way to keep yourself healthy, but sadly there will always be others (and perhaps the voice in your head is one of them) who will view you as weak, needy or broken for going to therapy. They aren't right. It's not the truth. Seeking out therapy is a sign of strength and an incredibly brave thing to do.

One of the magical things I am learning through therapy is that if people look at me differently because I am honest about the fact that I am not perfect, well, that's their problem not mine.

Been there, done that, it didn't work

My frankly rather terrible first few experiences of therapy burned me for many years. But it was wrong for me to write off all therapy and therapists based on some initial not-so-wonderful experiences.

Sure, if we've tried something before and it hasn't worked it's super tempting to think we know better and to give up, but not all therapy and not all therapists are the same. Once I clicked with therapy and found someone who showed me how it's meant to feel, I realised therapy is a process and it's very normal for there to be a certain amount of trial and error that goes on before you find what works for you. Which means that it's perfectly possible and even quite likely that you might have to test a few people out before deciding to commit to one.

But I'm OK... ish

The feeling of not deserving help is all too common. Whatever scary thoughts, panic attacks or deep, bone-penetrating sadness I experience must be normal because I don't have any 'real' problems to complain about. I'd tell myself, 'Your life isn't falling apart, so if you *feel* like you're falling apart, then you are the one who is wrong. Just effing deal with it Jo.'

But the thing about feelings is that they aren't wrong, nor are they right for that matter. They are just (very real and important) indicators of what's going on below the surface. So, it doesn't matter if your life circumstances are objectively better or worse than other people who may or may not be coping, if YOU are feeling something you don't understand or can't manage, you can get some help with that.

I'd be wasting their time

Despite cognitively knowing it is better to seek help before we're so far gone we're almost lost, we still feel guilty when we seek treatment, as if we are stealing it from someone who needs it more. These feelings can be even more acute for those of us living in the UK with the overstretched, under-resourced NHS. But here's the thing – there is no set 'rule' about how bad things need to be before you can seek support, even in the context of the NHS.

I have it on good authority from therapists working within the UK healthcare system that if you go to your GP and say you're not doing great and would like to explore therapy, they will refer you to a local team of psychologists and other therapists providing psychological therapy for mild to moderate mental health difficulties, including anxiety and depression (see page 190). It's very important to know *you won't be turned away*.

From experience, when accessing therapy privately and through insurance and employee assistance programmes (EAPs – more on these schemes on page 201), you are likely to have some sort of initial assessment to determine the level of care you need before either starting with your therapist or them helping you find who is best placed to support you, but by no means will you be turned away and not offered any kind of help or support.

There are of course occasions when a therapist might not be able to work with you or will suggest an alternative therapist, for a variety of reasons, such as they don't have the capacity, skill, time or expertise to help you. They may also have a conflict of interest or another reason it would be unethical for them to take you on as a client, such as:

▶ *You have close connections with their existing clients.* If the therapist can see that the connection between you and an existing client might raise issues of confidentiality, they wouldn't be able to see both clients.

▶ *Counter-transference is at play.* This is where the therapist's own past could potentially interfere with their support. It could be that your looks, personality, mannerisms or issues remind them of someone or something they are still working on.

▶ *Conflicts in personal or religious beliefs* (see page 250).

▶ *Mutual friends or family.* Interacting with your therapist outside of therapy doesn't help with maintaining healthy boundaries, so if they know they have a shared connection with you they would be unlikely to take you on as a client.

It's worth bearing in mind that therapists might not always tell you the reason for the conflict of interest, or even that there is one. This can be a bit annoying and frustrating to be on the receiving end of; however it's also reassuring to know if a therapist doesn't take you on as a client it is likely not to be personal.

It's too expensive

There's no denying it, it sure can be pricey going to therapy privately, but as we'll see in Chapter Ten, there are many ways to access therapy that are either free or at a low price point that many people either don't know about or don't explore (see page 201).

TELLING OTHERS

One of the first things many of us have to tackle when we find ourselves having therapy is how we tell people in our lives that we are doing so. For some of us this will be a bigger deal than for others. It also might vary depending on who you are confiding in; for example you might feel totally comfortable telling your friends you're in therapy, but less so your old-fashioned grandparents or new boss.

The very first thing I'd say is there is absolutely nothing wrong with going to therapy and there is nothing wrong with you for seeking support from therapy. You would never criticise someone for studying to improve their knowledge of a subject, and therapy is a kind of education in yourself and a way to improve your knowledge of you. If you feel comfortable telling people you are in therapy, then go for it, but if you would rather keep that element of your life private, that is perfectly fine too.

As scary as it might seem to tell someone you're in therapy, I promise you the vast majority of people will support you. However, there are some people who do not support the idea of therapy at all, seeing it as a sign of weakness, rather than a path to self-improvement. When I first told my parents I was seeing someone back at university, it is safe to say I was not met with the wave of support I had hoped for. Looking back now, I can see they were probably more than likely fearful of what that meant for me, and perhaps more than a little in denial about the state of my mental health. But at the time I didn't know what to think or feel, other than a deep shame, so I clammed up and decided that I shouldn't bring up the topic again with them.

REASONS TO TALK ABOUT YOUR THERAPY

▶ *Reassuring family and friends*. Contrary to how my family reacted, it could very well be that your friends and family have worried about your mental health for a while, and therefore telling them you are in therapy could act as a helpful reassurance for them of your progress.

▶ *Setting clear expectations*. If people close to you are aware of your therapy, they will have a forewarning about potential upcoming lifestyle or behaviour changes. For instance, if you start implementing a new way of doing certain things your family members can support you with that choice. I always find it helpful to say 'My therapist has suggested I try...' even if it is something we came to together.

▶ *Building your support system*. Having strong support around you definitely speeds up the recovery process. The motivating factor alone of having your very own cheerleading squad is very powerful.

▶ *Creating accountability and commitment*. Once you tell someone you are in therapy, it reconfirms that you are committed to the process. It's similar to having a workout buddy at the gym – it's someone to keep you accountable.

▶ *Becoming comfortable with the process*. If you still feel uncomfortable about being in therapy, talking to a supportive friend could help you see there is nothing to be ashamed of.

▶ *Avoiding confusion about your whereabouts.*
You might find you simply have to tell people in your life about your therapy as they need to know where you are, like your boss if you're disappearing early every Tuesday or your partner if you're getting home late every Thursday.

▶ *Helping others overcome their struggles.*
If your experience in therapy can help someone else, talk to them about it. Use your growth to encourage growth in others.

This last point is a big one and something I've found rings true time and time again. It probably helps that I talk about my therapy so freely these days with everyone, from my mum, my neighbours and parents at the school gates to thousands on the Internet, but I can't count the heart-warming number of people who have reached out and told me they would never have gone and sought therapy had they not heard me talking about it. This is incredible. And even more incredibly, and very much to my surprise, my own therapy-mistrusting mother very recently sought therapy to help her with a particular issue she was going through at the time. I almost fell off my chair when she asked me how she would go about talking to someone!

REASONS NOT TO TALK ABOUT YOUR THERAPY

▶ *External validation.* If you are telling people about going to therapy with the sole aim of bragging about your self-improvement then I'm sorry but I think that kind of defeats the purpose. Your satisfaction should be the focus of your therapy, not someone else's.

▶ *A negative support system.* If telling people about your therapy could slow down or derail your progress, consider discussing it only after your recovery.

▶ *You need time to get stronger.* It may take time to build your self-esteem before discussing your therapy with others. You need to get to a place where you can feel confident about your journey, no matter what anyone says about it.

▶ *You're just not comfortable with it.* If you're not ready to tell people about your therapy, trust your instincts. This is something that you're doing for yourself, and there is nothing wrong with keeping it personal.

HOW MUCH THERAPY DO I NEED?

Sadly, there's no set formula that a therapist can apply to tell you that for your depression, for example, you will need exactly 10 sessions with them and after that all will be peachy. It just doesn't work like that. Other factors, such as what you are looking to get out of therapy, what type of therapy you're having and what type of person you are, will also come into play. Some people find a short course of therapy is more than enough to help support them with whatever it is they are dealing with, while others will want or need longer-term support over a number of months or years. Some therapies are much more directive and rapid, others unfold at a slower pace. Essentially it all depends!

That said, a couple of sessions probably isn't quite enough to really get into any issues in a meaningful way – you'll both still be trying to get to know each other. As we'll see in Chapter Eleven, for the first few sessions the therapist will be in assessment mode, gathering information about you, asking questions before pulling together ideas about what might be going on for you and what might help. You'll also still be in the process of opening up and establishing trust.

Anecdotally, I hear from my therapist friends that a very general rule of thumb is most people see a therapist for roughly 6–20 sessions. Harley Therapy data tell us the average length of the therapy–client relationship they have seen since they started recording data in 2017 is just over six sessions. Interestingly, the UK National Institute for Health and Care Excellence (NICE) guidelines for moderate to severe depression suggest that NHS Trusts offer patients 16–20 sessions of therapy. Very often there will be clear goals you will be working towards together with your therapist, regular reviews of those goals and discussions about how much more therapy you might need.

But how long is too long? Some people worry that seeing a therapist long term can create an unhealthy dependency (see page 249), but as someone who has currently had therapy weekly over four years, I now know that long-term therapy is more about having the time to take things slowly, build up trust and explore complex issues rather than a reliance on and an inability to grow without it. I find it very healing in itself to have therapy with someone I trust to accept and respect me. Over the years, I've found therapy isn't just about resolving one-off issues for me. Rather, it's about having a regular time and place to prioritise my mental health and well-being. However, it can still be useful even in long-term therapy to set goals, particularly when you've seen someone for a long time, as sessions can sometimes drift (see page 210 for more on this).

HELPING OTHERS TO GET THERAPY

What if you know someone who might need help and you don't know how to help them do this? You might feel frustrated or powerless in this situation, especially as we've seen that being pressured into therapy isn't ideal. However, if you're close to that person, you may be well-placed to get them a step closer to therapy. I've gently helped a few people in my life reach out to get therapy and here's what I'd say about doing this:

Don't force them
As we've already heard, you really shouldn't pressure someone to get support. All you can do is gently try to encourage them.

One way I've found to do this is by bringing the conversation back to you and your own more positive experiences of therapy. This was especially helpful with my mum, who was very distrustful of therapy, but by slowly normalising my own therapy and making it personal it seemed to take some of the stigma and embarrassment away for her when she reached out for support. For example, I might casually mention going to a therapy appointment when chatting about my day – not the detail of its content, but I'd say things like 'After therapy I did X, Y, Z' or 'Can you watch Bella today while I have therapy?' – to the more obvious sharing practical tips in conversation, such as 'Oh, you know, when I feel like that my therapist has suggested trying A, B or C.'

Frame it with care

It really does help to start the conversation by letting the other person know how much you care about them, even (or maybe especially) if they're doing something that's causing you stress. This sounds like a blindingly obvious thing to say, but often we can be so focused on the solution that we don't stop to think about how the message is coming across to the other person. 'I think you need to see someone' is such a loaded phrase and can be very hard to hear, however kindly it is delivered, so compassion should always be at the forefront of our minds when discussing this topic with our loved ones, especially if you can see very clearly how much the other person needs the support and help.

Reassure them about privacy

It's a huge misconception about therapy that a lot of people believe that if they tell a therapist something, it's going to somehow get out. I've had to explicitly tell people in my life that, other than for a handful of reasons, this simply isn't the case (see page 213).

Look after yourself

You might have seen it – there's an Internet meme that says 'I'm in therapy to deal with the people in my life who won't go to therapy'. Although it's supposed to be funny, boy has it got a lot of truth to it. If everyone in our lives had therapy, the beneficial ripple effect would be rather wonderful, but let's be honest, the likelihood of that happening is pretty slim. As much as we'd like to, we cannot force somebody else to get help. Ultimately, it's their own decision, it's not up to us. Therefore, at some point, we have to protect ourselves. At the very least, setting boundaries with someone will give us some peace of mind. After all, we are the only people we can control.

Therapy thoughts

Jonny Benjamin MBE, award-winning mental health campaigner, film producer, public speaker and author of *The Stranger on the Bridge*, shared with me the biggest lesson he's learned from therapy: '*It takes time! I've always wanted a quick fix. Who doesn't? But patience and persistence are so vital in therapy.*'

Chapter Ten

HOW TO FIND THE RIGHT

Therapy for You

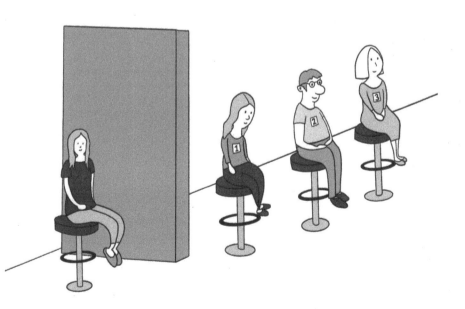

There are hundreds, if not thousands, of different types of therapy out there, which is great as it means help is definitely available, but knowing which to pick can feel more than a little overwhelming.

NICE recommends certain therapies for certain difficulties, such as CBT, which is used to help a range of concerns including depression, anxiety, obsessive compulsive disorder (OCD), managing long-term illnesses, eating disorders, PTSD and schizophrenia. But other therapies might work for you just as well.

All therapies do have certain things in common, such as they are all ways of understanding how someone ticks and what might help them change. And many therapists will actually draw on different approaches at any given time – even within the same session they might use a variety of techniques and methodologies.

Here's a high-level look at some of the more common types of therapy to help you decide which might be best suited to you:

HUMANISTIC THERAPY

Humanistic therapies focus on the individual as a whole and put the client at the centre of the approach. They use a range of theories and practices to help you understand your thoughts and feelings. A humanistic therapist will work to create a safe, supportive space where clients will be able to explore themselves and their potential, ultimately working towards developing their own personal growth – mentally, emotionally and spiritually. You'll likely spend time exploring ways to grow and increase self-acceptance along with discussing the issues you're dealing with.

There are many different types of humanistic therapy such as Gestalt therapy, person- /client-centred therapy, transactional analysis and transpersonal therapy, with person-centred therapy being one of the most widely used approaches to therapy for decades.

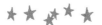

Humanistic therapy might be right for you if... you are feeling lost, struggling with low self-esteem, have relationship issues or are generally looking to improve your well-being. Humanistic therapy covers such a broad range of therapeutic methods, it could benefit many mental health concerns. It would suit someone interested in exploring their life and their issues from a wide range of angles. Humanistic therapists will also work with people living with many specific conditions, such as anxiety, addiction, depression, OCD, and more.

From the Other Chair
PERSON-CENTRED THERAPY

As Kemi Omijeh (@therapy_with_kemi on Instagram), London-based therapist, explains, the person-centred approach to counselling and psychotherapy was developed in the forties and fifties by the American psychologist Carl Rogers, who argued that when clients are able to 'direct' the therapy themselves, they generally make better progress than when the session is led by the therapist.

Person-centred therapy emphasises the quality of the relationship between the client and therapist, seeing this as the most important mechanism helping a client to change. Like most therapeutic approaches, it does not involve being given advice or being told what to do by someone else. The person-centred therapist's aim is to facilitate self-reflection, and help the client learn to trust themselves and realise their own potential.

The therapist is there to encourage and support the client and to guide the therapeutic process without interrupting or interfering with the client's process of self-discovery.

The person-centred approach sets out three core ingredients needed to be cultivated by the therapist in order to help their clients achieve growth in the therapy room. They sound simple when listed out, but in fact take many years of training to achieve. They are:

1   The therapist must be completely genuine (also known as 'congruence').

2   The therapist must strive to understand the client's experience (or 'empathy').

3   The therapist must accept the client non-judgementally and unconditionally (known as having 'unconditional positive regard').

COGNITIVE BEHAVIOURAL THERAPY (CBT)

CBT is a type of short-term, usually time-limited, therapy focused on changing how you relate to your thoughts and how those thoughts affect your behaviour in the here and now, rather than looking too much into the past. It combines cognitive therapy (examining the things you think) and behaviour therapy (examining the things you do). It is a problem-solving, solution-based therapy, as opposed to spending lots of time talking things through. In CBT a therapist will help you identify thinking and behaviour patterns that aren't working for you and give you healthy alternatives and skills you can practise in your own life, teaching you coping skills for dealing with different issues.

CBT might be right for you if... you are dealing with an anxiety disorder, panic attacks, bipolar disorder or depression. It is ideal for anyone who wants clear goals and practical techniques.

DIALECTICAL BEHAVIOUR THERAPY (DBT)

DBT is actually a specific type of CBT, focused on practical ways to regulate emotions and skills to help you take responsibility for unhealthy or disruptive behaviour. It is based on teaching problem-solving techniques and learning acceptance strategies.

DBT might be right for you if... other types of therapy haven't worked for you so far. DBT is typically used to help people with certain personality disorders, chronic suicidal ideations, PTSD or eating disorders.

From the Other Chair
BEREAVEMENT COUNSELLING

As Sasha Bates, psychotherapist and author of *Languages of Loss*, explains, bereavement counselling is a type of targeted counselling intended specifically for the bereaved. While grief is a natural response to losing someone you care about, some of the huge emotions can feel overwhelming. You may feel safer having a supportive and experienced other person alongside as you go through these unfamiliar feelings, to help you understand that whatever reactions you are having are not unusual. You may feel you don't want to burden your friends or that there is a time limit on how much, how often or how long you grieve for, which is not the case. Grief is individual and it may affect you in different ways at different times. You may want help if your emotions are so intense you feel you can't go on, or if you can't cope with your day-to-day life, for example, if you struggle to go to work, look after children or socialise with friends. If you're experiencing these feelings, it's important to get support.

Accessing bereavement counselling or therapy is done in largely the same ways as general emotional support (see below for more on this). Most counsellors and therapists will be happy to support you with bereavement. However, as always, it's best to check with them if you're not sure. Many hospices, for example Marie Curie Hospices, have bereavement support services for families (see page 262). This is usually available for close family and friends of people who have received hospice care. How much support a hospice is able to give will depend on their resources.

PSYCHODYNAMIC THERAPY

Often psychodynamic therapy is mistaken for psychoanalysis (see below). The idea in psychodynamic therapy is to talk through your past experiences and feelings to improve self-awareness and change old patterns. In this technique, your therapist will want to get to know your feelings, beliefs and life experiences to help you recognise and change reoccurring patterns. It can be used in both the short term (over a few months) or as a longer-term therapy (over a few years).

Psychodynamic therapy might be right for you if... you're generally all right, but are struggling with your past and how it may be affecting your future. That said, psychodynamic therapy can be used to treat any number of issues and may often be woven into other techniques.

PSYCHOANALYTIC THERAPY

Psychoanalysis is what most people think of when they hear the term 'talking therapy', where a patient lies on a couch talking to a Freud-like figure for hours at a time. It's been around for years and is still a very common form of therapy. It can be very useful for bringing unconscious problems to the surface to be dissected and resolved.

Psychoanalytic therapy might be right for you if... you have anxiety or self-esteem issues you want to explore further.

From the Other Chair
EYE MOVEMENT DESENSITISATION AND REPROCESSING THERAPY (EMDR)

As Laura Bethel, psychotherapist and EMDR specialist, explains, EMDR therapy is a psychotherapy technique that uses bilateral stimulation, usually with eye movements, to reduce the physical reactions associated with traumatic memories. It lessens the emotional intensity of difficult and challenging memories, helping to change negative beliefs and lessen distress by enabling the brain to reprocess memories properly.

As a therapeutic approach, EMDR is based on the model of Adaptive Information Processing. Along with Trauma-Focused CBT, it is recognised by the World Health Organization as a treatment for PTSD, but can be used to help with a range of other mental illnesses and issues such as depression, addictions, anxiety, relationship issues and also more serious illnesses such as psychosis and aspects of personality disorders.

EMDR has a very specific structure and format that requires specialised skills in order for it to be delivered safely and therefore it should only be carried out by trained and skilled practitioners.

The above list is just a flavour of some of the many therapies out there. But even after just reading this short list it might feel a bit overwhelming to commit to a specific kind of therapy. I have found it helpful to keep in mind that many therapists integrate a number of different techniques from various types of therapy, taking the pressure off having to commit to one specific type. And it also comes down to personal preference. Much of the research into therapy shows that the relationship with your therapist is often one of the biggest drivers of change and I have personally found this to be the case.

Try not to place too much pressure on yourself, and remember it's perfectly normal to try one approach, find that it doesn't work for you and then try another.

WHAT DOES THERAPY FEEL LIKE?

This can't easily be answered as it depends on a whole host of things. Therapy will feel different depending on the type of therapy, the therapist and what you're like as an individual. For me, therapy can feel:

- comforting, but also at times wildly uncomfortable
- like a non-judgemental space, but without a doubt can still hold me to account
- safe, but also at times I can feel a little attacked
- like I'm tied up in knots, but it can also help me feel a little less tangled

FORMS OF THERAPY

In addition to the different types of therapy, there are also many different forms that therapy can take. Below are just a few:

Individual
This is the most common type of therapy. All therapy will be one-on-one unless otherwise stated.

Group
The vast majority of group therapy deals with some form of substance abuse or addiction, but that is not to say it will all be addiction-focused. Group therapy can also be useful for many other things including trauma and grief, and for victims of physical abuse.

Couples
Often people think going to couples therapy is a sign that their relationship has failed or is failing, but in reality it can actually be an incredibly healthy tool for developing a deeper bond or preparing for changes ahead. Many couples find enormous value in this type of therapy when responsibilities shift, perhaps due to a change in finances or becoming parents.

Family
Family therapy can be valuable for all familial relationships, whether between siblings, parents and children, other family members or indeed any group of people who care about each other and call each other 'family'.

Life events

Some therapists will specialise in very specific life moments including, but not limited to, money or medical issues, childbirth, divorce, death, impotence and infertility.

Online/telephone therapy

It's becoming more and more common for therapists to offer remote services via phone or video chat. If special situations prevent you from seeing a therapist in an office, this may be a great choice.

I have been writing this book during the COVID-19 pandemic and, as such, there could hardly be a more appropriate time to be talking about online support. I have been unable to access face-to-face support for months now. Instead, like so many others during this time, my therapy sessions have taken place virtually via my laptop or phone in my kitchen, living room, car, and even my bedroom. We've been interrupted by barking dogs, postmen, husbands being locked out, children wailing their hungry or bored requests from other rooms, Wi-Fi issues and much more. A world away from the sanctuary of the therapy room! And, to begin with, I'll admit, I didn't like it at all – seeing myself on screen, the unfamiliar digital space hanging between us, the constant distractions, it all felt really odd. But as the weeks and months have worn on we've made it work and, instead of feeling distanced from my therapist, I have been surprised to find the opposite to be true. If anything, tackling these issues together, learning how to make it work, sharing a little more of my world with her and seeing a little glimpse into hers, has actually helped me feel far closer to her. Online therapy, it turns out, provides a sense of intimacy and closeness I hadn't anticipated.

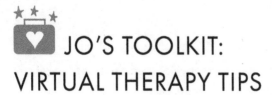

JO'S TOOLKIT: VIRTUAL THERAPY TIPS

▶ Awkward is OK. No matter what platform your therapist is using and however tech-savvy they are, it's still going to be a different experience from in-person, so don't be alarmed if it doesn't feel like you and your therapist are 'in sync' right away. Let your therapist take the lead if you feel weird, or voice it out loud to them as often just saying it can help you get more comfortable.

▶ Remember, if you've swapped from in-person to online, it's normal to 'grieve' the loss of in-person support.

▶ If you're meeting your therapist for the first time online, be patient, it might take just a little longer for this 2D experience to feel more 3D.

▶ Try to find a quiet, private, comfortable spot where you won't be interrupted, with good phone reception or Wi-Fi.

▶ Use headphones for more privacy.

▶ Have a glass of water and tissues nearby.

▶ It can be really distracting looking at yourself. There's usually an option that allows you to minimise yourself, but if the platform you're using doesn't have it or you can't find it, you can always put a Post-it over yourself. We just aren't used to seeing ourselves in the therapy chair.

▶ Try not to sit in front of a window as this makes it harder for the therapist to see you.

▶ Lean into the unique benefits. There are some things you can do with online therapy that you can't necessarily do in person. For example, it's probably not appropriate to bring your cat to an in-person therapy session, but introducing your therapist to your furry friend is more than acceptable and is likely to enhance your connection as they see and learn more about you.

Having experienced a number of different approaches and forms over the years, I have a rough idea of what kind of therapy works for me, but I'd still say the type and form of therapy is actually less important than whether the therapist's way of working feels right for you. And realistically, the only way you'll know this is by giving it a try and seeing what works.

HOW TO FIND THE RIGHT THERAPIST

There are hundreds of therapists out there from various prof-essional backgrounds, such as psychotherapists, psychologists, coaches, psychoanalysts, counsellors or psychiatrists, and they all have their own unique personal style. Some therapists train in more than one kind of therapy and may decide to combine a few approaches if that will help you best.

It's worth remembering that the term 'therapist' is not regulated, which means absolutely anyone can call themselves a therapist without any qualifications whatsoever. This means it is really important to always check that someone has the appropriate qualifications to be offering you the type of therapy that they are – there's a little more about how you can do this below.

But first, how do you actually find a therapist? There are a few ways to do this in the UK:

▶ through the NHS

▶ privately

▶ through your employer or educational setting

▶ through insurance

▶ through charities/third sector

The NHS

In the UK most people's first port of call when looking to access therapy through the NHS is to speak to their GP. If you express an interest in talking therapy, your GP will then refer you for support via your local Improving Access to Psychological Therapies (IAPT) team. These are teams of psychologists and other therapists providing psychological talking therapy for mild to moderate mental health difficulties, including anxiety and depression.

What many people don't know is that the majority of IAPT services have their own websites where you can self-refer directly without having to see your GP at all. The best way to find yours is to google 'IAPT [your local area]'. It is very important to stress that you DO NOT need to have a diagnosed mental health issue to refer yourself to IAPT. It might be that you're experiencing stress, anxiety, phobias, having nightmares, feeling low or finding it hard to cope with work, life or relationships. That said, if you have already been diagnosed with a mental health concern that's also not a barrier and you can still refer yourself to IAPT directly.

I have it on good authority from NHS therapists that

someone from the IAPT service will then get in touch, usually within a few weeks. They'll ask you for more details about what you're experiencing, which is known as an assessment, and if they think they can help you, they'll recommend a form of therapy for you. This is based on your symptoms and how severe they are, and consists of guided self-help with a therapist to support you, CBT or depression counselling. Waiting times for the first session vary, but the service should tell you what to expect.

According to the NHS, 75 per cent of people referred to local IAPT services should start treatment within 6 weeks of a referral, and 95 per cent should start treatment within 18 weeks of a referral, but it's sadly true that some people have to wait much longer.

It might be that you require a more specialist service than what IAPT can offer, usually known as 'secondary care services' (which essentially means that they work with people with more complex or long-standing needs). These services may cover a range of different issues, such as eating disorders, perinatal mental health issues, personality disorders or trauma.

Private therapy

I recently had a single friend tell me that looking for a therapist privately, especially online, is a little like the modern dating process. Seriously! She recognised parallels with this process and trying to find dates on Tinder. Now I'm not saying it's exactly like dating, but there are definitely some similarities between the two in that you are looking at photos and reading bios to find 'the one', which might mean having to try a few out, which could be quite frustrating, but ultimately worth it in the long run.

Ask for recommendations

Asking for recommendations from friends, family members or a doctor you trust can be a really good place to start looking for a therapist. It's also a good way to open up and ease into a conversation about mental health.

There are a couple of things to consider first if you ask for recommendations. First, if the person recommending their therapist to you is a close family member or friend it is likely the therapist will not be able to take you on as a client on ethical grounds if they also currently see your connection (see page 176). Secondly, even if they aren't a close acquaintance is there any chance you might talk about this particular person in therapy, possibly in a negative way? Because even though the therapist will do what they can to stay completely neutral, even just knowing they see this person too could jeopardise you feeling your therapist is entirely unbiased, and make you uncomfortable, possibly harming your trust. Finally, everyone is so unique and what they need from therapy and their therapist can be vastly different. Knowing this and knowing how important the relationship is to the therapeutic process, I'm always a little hesitant to recommend my therapist to other people. And when I do, it always comes with the caveat of 'I think she's brilliant and she's really helped me, but you may well disagree.'

Online

Most people search for a private therapist online, but it can be more than a little confusing to know where to start.

It's a good idea to only ever use reliable websites that only list therapists who are registered with a professional body. That way, you can have peace of mind that your therapist is a qualified professional. See page 262 for a list of professional bodies.

Employer/educational setting

Some employers provide free counselling for their employees, called employee assistance programmes (EAPs), which can provide you with short-term mental health care, referrals and financial advice. Ask your HR department to see if this is something your company offers. This is particularly important to tap into if your difficulties are making it hard for you to attend or return to work. I have also heard of some workers' unions offering free therapy sessions. Of course, these are not always an option, but very often such schemes are not clearly promoted so it is worth doing some digging.

If you are in education, many people don't know that most colleges and universities offer free counselling to students who need it.

Insurance

If you have private medical insurance, either through work or separately, it is always worth checking whether mental health provisions are covered. If your policy does cover therapy, in my experience providers are likely to have their own list of preferred therapists. That said, I have found that you still have a certain amount of choice of who you pick, so see page 197 for advice on picking a therapist.

Charities/third sector

There are many charities and voluntary organisations out there supporting people in a huge variety of ways: specific mental health charities, those aimed at children and families, women-specific charities, charities for veterans, bereavement services... the list is endless. Some charities also offer discounted or free talking therapies or group support.

Your local IAPT service (see either page 198 for discussion or

262 for contact details) should normally have a list and be able to signpost you, or you could do a quick search online.

OTHER LOWER COST OPTIONS

If the cost of long-term therapy is too much, it might be worth (if possible) considering paying for an initial assessment session to think about what your difficulties are and if the therapist can make any recommendations for things you could try, or resources to tap into, or books to read. Although this may not feel ideal, it could be enough to make things more manageable until another option is available. Other options could include:

▶ Ask about sliding scales. Not all therapists do this, but there are some out there who have sliding fee scales depending on what you can afford. It's always worth asking.

▶ Ask about pro bono. Again, not all, but some therapists will take on a number of clients for free, so don't be afraid to ask if they have pro bono spots open.

▶ Investigate universities, colleges and some teaching hospitals. They usually have clinics where people training to be psychotherapists, counsellors, psychologists, social workers and family therapists, etc. will see people at a reduced rate or even for free in order to get on-the-job experience.

▶ Consider group therapy or peer support groups, which can be cheaper or free.

▶ Do some research on whether you might suit one of the many talk- or text-based therapy apps as these can often be quicker and cheaper alternatives to in-person therapy. However, always remember to use a reputable app that uses accredited professionals, and as boring as it sounds you probably want to pick one with robust privacy and confidentiality settings.

HOW TO PICK SOMEONE

OK, so you've decided to take the plunge privately or through your insurance. Here comes the tricky part: how do you actually narrow it down and pick someone? In order to do this, you might want to consider the following:

Do you have any preferences?

You might not think you do, and maybe you genuinely don't mind, but it's worth spending a little bit of time thinking about what kind of person you might be most comfortable with. Does their gender, presentation or sexual orientation matter to you? Would you like them to be of a similar age or have similar characteristics to you? Or would you prefer them to be older or younger? Maybe you want a therapist who will challenge you and light a fire under your butt, or maybe you're looking for a space just to talk and process things with an unbiased third party. Perhaps you'd like a therapist from the same culture, race, ethnicity or who holds the same or similar religious or spiritual beliefs as you. Maybe you want a therapist who reminds you of one of your parents or a mentor figure, or maybe you need a therapist who feels more like a peer and a friend. And there are practical considerations to bear in mind too; for example do you want to see someone in your lunch hour and therefore they would need to be based near your workplace, or will you see them before or after work and therefore someone based nearer your home might be better suited?

What do their bios say?

Most therapists will put some time into making sure their bios or websites reflect who they are as people and therapists. It's not completely foolproof, but I have found that I can often get a rough idea of whether they'll be a good match for me just based on how they choose to present themselves.

Make a shortlist

I really recommend making a shortlist and setting up phone consultations with each and see what responses you get. Even if you just talk to them for five minutes, their tone, style, manner or even something as simple as their voice may tell you more than you think. Plus it also means that when you do go for that scary first appointment, they don't feel like quite such a stranger. These calls will also help you to investigate a few things like who they are, their availability, cost, how many therapy sessions to expect and how they might be able to help you, but they should also help you determine if you feel comfortable.

Below are some questions you might want to ask a potential new therapist:

▶ How often will we have sessions?

▶ How long are the sessions?

▶ How much do you charge?

▶ What are your qualifications and expertise?

▶ What approaches do you use?

▶ What's your cancellation policy?

- Have you had experience in seeing clients with my issues/ from my culture/background/religion before?

- Can I contact you in between sessions?

Expect some therapists to be full or unavailable – try not to see this as a rejection or a setback.

Trust your instincts

Everyone needs to find their The One and, while I do believe there is more than one The One for each person, rather unhelpfully there is no blueprint for finding them as it will come down to lots of different factors that will be unique to each person. That said, finding someone you feel comfortable with should always come first and foremost. Not only is your therapist someone you'll be seeing frequently, but they're also someone you need to be comfortable feeling vulnerable around.

That said, I'd stress that it's really important not to get too bogged down with having an instantly incredible connection. Ultimately at this stage you are simply trying to work out if you might match and be able to open up to this person at some point in the future. That might take some time to show itself, but some positive signs are that you are able to have a comfortable conversational rapport, you get the impression that they genuinely care about understanding you, you get the sense that you're respected and have a feeling of safety.

On top of finding a therapist you feel comfortable around, it's really helpful to find someone who is at least familiar with issues that are important to you. Some therapists will list that kind of stuff in their bios, but always feel free to ask prospective therapists whether they feel equipped to help you.

Oh and always, always, always make sure they are registered with one of the professional bodies. A list of the main UK professional organisations can be found on page 262, but please do your own research as this list is not exhaustive.

A small side note on peer support: I am a big fan of peer support groups and organisations. They are usually free or low-cost and are normally extremely accessible, and are a brilliant way to heal alongside people who have literally walked in your shoes. But it's really important if you access these services that they are inclusive, collaborative, informed and reciprocal and, above all, that you feel safe and supported.

Therapy thoughts

Hope Virgo, leading eating disorder campaigner and author, explained to me, '*It takes ages for me to open up, and for some people I just can't. This has meant in the past I have stuck at therapy without realising that not everyone clicks. I wish I had known that from the outset so I could either hunt around for what I wanted or been able to ask.*'

Chapter Eleven
THE FIRST
Session

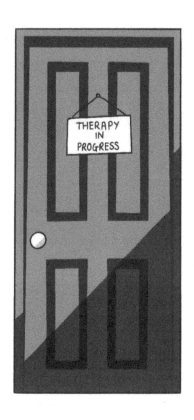

You've found a therapist you like the sound of, you've booked your first session with them, or got confirmation of your appointment, but what happens next? That limbo period in between making or receiving your appointment and turning up can be quite a nerve-racking time.

It's really very normal to feel anxious in the run up to starting therapy. Starting anything new brings with it an element of anticipation, whether that's nerves or excitement, or most likely a combination of the two.

But it's important to keep in mind that the hardest part – the bit you had to do alone – is over. From now on, you will have your therapist to help guide you through the rest. So take this time before your first session to give yourself a break and be proud of yourself for making the conscious decision to bring about positive changes in your life.

There's no need to prepare anything for your first therapy session if you don't feel like it. Just rocking up is totally fine. However, taking a moment or two to check in with yourself and getting clear on a few things can help you get the most out of your session.

Here are a few ideas you might like to try:

Reflect on what you want from therapy
First up, it could help to have a bit of a think around what you're looking to get out of therapy. This could provide you with a direction for your sessions and also set you up with a starting point to chart your progress along the way.

What are my goals?
Everyone's goals from therapy will be different, such as 'feel better', 'stop having the same fight with my partner', 'heal my depression', 'find healthier ways to cope with stress' or maybe just

'feel differently'. Whatever your goals might be, communicate them to your therapist!

When I went to my first session with my current therapist I took in a list of all the things that worked and didn't work for me in therapy and all the things I wanted to get out of it, as well as some of the topics I wanted to dig into further with her. I felt a little silly taking a list with me, but she didn't bat an eyelid and it really helped me to focus on the key points I wanted to get across rather than try to get everything out all at once.

Think about timings

You might find it helpful to block out some time before and after your session. Beforehand you will probably want to give yourself a little cushion of time just to make sure you find the place OK without rushing and have some time to breathe and calm your nerves. Afterwards it can be really helpful not to have to suddenly rush back to your 'normal' life (see page 117 on what I call 'therapy hangovers').

What to take with you

People often wonder about what they should take to therapy. Your therapy is all about you, so really you just need to take yourself. But also because of this, you can take whatever you need to feel comfortable, whether that's a bottle of water, a toy to fiddle with or your dog (although you might want to check with your therapist first on this one – however, speaking from personal experience, having my dog in the therapy room is a hugely comforting, although occasionally distracting, experience).

Give yourself a break

Last but certainly not least would be to give yourself a huge pat on the back for taking this leap. Yes, it's nerve-racking, but it takes a huge amount of courage to agree to meet with a stranger and share your innermost world with them. You've taken the first massive step, and you deserve to celebrate that.

WHAT ACTUALLY HAPPENS IN THE FIRST SESSION?

Every first session I've ever had has been different, but there have been a few things they've all had in common. It's good to bear in mind that, all being well, this is likely to be the first of many sessions and a fair chunk of this first one will likely revolve around boring admin stuff, as well as your therapist getting a feel for you as their new client.

Here's a little bit about what exactly you might experience:

Housekeeping

Every first session with a new therapist will involve a certain amount of housekeeping. These tasks will vary depending on the therapist and the circumstances, but might include such things as taking care of insurance and billing information, if applicable. They will likely spend some time explaining the process of therapy and in particular the way they work. They will also discuss confidentiality with you. And there will inevitably be some forms for you to fill in, such as your contact details, maybe a confidentiality agreement, some information about them perhaps, and your therapist might even ask you to take some paperwork away and answer some questions before the next session.

CONFIDENTIALITY:

When they will share information and when they won't...

Trust and confidentiality sit at the very heart of an effective therapeutic relationship. This means you can speak to your therapist knowing that your friends, family, work colleagues and so on will not get to learn what you have said in your sessions and neither will your therapist's friends, family, work colleagues and so on.

However, therapists can discuss your care with a strictly limited number of other professionals for sound ethical reasons. These are:

▶ *Supervision.* Therapists discuss clients regularly with their own supervisor (another experienced therapist), but the supervisor is also under a duty to maintain confidentiality, so any information about you will be treated confidentially. In the UK, it's seen as unethical for a therapist to work without supervision because it helps your therapist look after their own mental health, so they're better able to support you, and it means someone else is aware of how your therapist is treating you, to make sure it's appropriate.

▶ *Safety.* If your therapist is concerned that you're at serious risk of harming yourself or someone else, they may need to inform your GP, a healthcare professional or someone else. They should tell you first if they're going to do this.

▶ *Organisational confidentiality.* If your therapist is part of a GP practice, for example, confidentiality could apply to the practice as a whole rather than to the individual therapist. This may mean that information is available to your GP. Again, your therapist should tell you if this is the case.

The nitty-gritty

The first session is usually pretty guided by the therapist in an attempt to get to know you and what you are experiencing. Depending on the therapist and their approach to therapy, you might be asked questions about your childhood, education, job, relationships, thoughts, feelings or actions. Your responses will help your therapist understand you and work out how best to help you.

It's often said that the first appointment is more helpful to the therapist than it is to the client, and as a result the session can sometimes feel a little disappointing or frustrating if you don't know that's what's going to happen. However, that doesn't mean you can't get a lot from it too.

Be as open as you can

It's hard to open up, especially when we have only just met someone and we are a little unsure of what to say or how to act. After all, most of us spend our days not thinking too much about our feelings, so to suddenly start probing can feel a little uncomfortable. You can talk about as much or as little during the first session as you're comfortable with. But either way, the therapist will expect to talk a little bit at the least about your history and what has brought you to therapy. Try to stick with it as much as you can, even if it feels a bit tough. Being open to exploring the uncomfortable bits is often where the most progress is made. That said, don't feel you have to cover absolutely everything in that first session. Trust is something that takes time to build. Plus, you're going to miss things and that's perfectly OK – it will all come out over time if it's important, and your therapist will be there to help you share in your own time.

Ask questions

As well as talking to your therapist about what your goals might be and what you're looking to get out of therapy, this is also your chance to ask any questions you might have. Don't feel awkward about this – they will be expecting it and it's unlikely you will be asking them anything that someone else hasn't asked before.

Listen to your gut

You've probably worked out by now that finding the right fit for you is a big part of finding a therapist. However, this doesn't mean that you have to instantly 'click' with them or even that they have to be your very favourite person, or that they won't challenge you. It means that you feel safe, accepted and heard with them. Take note during the session of how they made you feel. Did you feel comfortable opening up to them? Did they express things to you clearly in a way that made sense to you? It's a hard thing to try to put your finger on, but did you feel heard, understood and respected? Could you see yourself opening up to them and sharing the deep and difficult things in your life? Is there anything about them that makes you feel like your guard is up when you're with them?

What you're looking for is someone who strikes a nice balance between challenging you and making you feel secure and understood. It's true that therapy can sometimes feel uncomfortable while navigating difficult emotions and experiences. But it's important you feel like you're making strides towards feeling better too. If that's not happening, make sure you take into consideration your doubts, trust yourself and move on to the next. Somewhere out there is The One, and the likelihood is, like lots of great love affairs, you need to listen to your gut and go with your instincts to find them.

JO'S TOOLKIT: SIGNS THEY MIGHT BE A GOOD FIT

▶ You feel comfortable.

▶ You feel hopeful.

▶ You feel heard and understood.

▶ They answer your questions openly and honestly.

▶ They empower you in your decision on choosing your therapist, rather than making you feel you *have* to pick them.

▶ You feel like they are the kind of person you will be able to open up to.

▶ They feel competent to help you.

▶ You are (even if it's only a little bit) excited about getting started!

You can swap

It's *totally* OK to swap therapists! Remember, you are the one in charge – if something feels off, you have no obligation to keep seeing them. A professional therapist will not take your decision to see someone else personally and if the relationship isn't working, chances are they probably feel it too. They will want you to get the most out of therapy, if not with them, then with someone else. And although it can be awkward as hell, it is, however, always worth discussing this with your therapist before walking out of the door in case it is something that can be worked on.

Even under NHS care, you can ask to swap and I've been reliably informed by therapists working in the NHS that you will *not* go back to the bottom of the waiting list. Having said that, you might have to wait for the next therapist to become available, but rest assured, this won't be as long as going to the back of the queue.

Remember, you are doing a hard, brave thing and you deserve supportive mental health care. It's tricky to find the right therapist, so try not to put too much pressure on yourself; it might be a hard thing, but it's a hard thing that's definitely worth doing for yourself.

Give it a few sessions

Progress and getting to know and trust someone take time, so unless the therapist has been enormously unprofessional or rude, or you've felt unsafe, uncomfortable or unwelcome, try to give it a few sessions to work out whether they are indeed right for you or not.

That said, don't be afraid to push back if something doesn't feel right to you, and if something *really* doesn't feel right, you're under no obligation to continue seeing someone. Therapy won't always feel amazing, but it should always feel safe.

Feeling awkward is perfectly normal

Most people will experience a few awkward stumbling blocks or silences in therapy at some point, it's all part of the journey and even more likely in the first session. But be assured that your therapist is likely the very best person to deal with this and will have plenty of practice on being on the other side, to the point where it might feel awkward to you but it's very unlikely to be awkward for them.

Feeling nervous is perfectly normal

Nerves are not only OK, they are very normal. It might help calm the nerves to keep in mind that it's not your job to keep the conversation flowing or perfectly articulate your feelings. The hope is that, with a good therapist, over time they'll be able to help you find the words to talk about what's going on and make sense of things. A good therapist will hold up a mirror and help you find your own path, in your own way, in a supportive and healing manner. There are no stupid things to say, no right way of being. My therapist says, 'it's all relevant'.

BEYOND THE FIRST SESSION

You might find you leave your first session with more questions, thoughts or random concerns than answers. And that's pretty normal and totally OK. Below are a few things I wish someone had told me a long time ago.

Who is supposed to talk first?

There are no set rules on who speaks first; it usually depends on the particular therapist and their style – some will wait for you to talk first, while others will say something like, 'Is there anything you'd like to talk about today?' Most therapists, whether they speak first or not, will let you lead the conversation in whatever direction you'd like it to go. In general, it is you, and not your therapist, who is in charge of how you spend the session so most will wait for you to talk first. Remember, there's no set formula when it comes to chatting to a therapist, so try to follow your instincts on where you might want to begin and things should flow from there.

Will they take notes?

All therapists will make notes, but not all will do so during the session. In fact, the vast majority of therapists I have seen have not made any notes during our sessions.

If your therapist does make notes while you are sat there, it's unlikely they will be taking down everything you say verbatim and much more likely that they're just jotting a few things down to help them write their case notes afterwards or so they can refer back to important details in the future.

Will they diagnose me?

Clinical psychologists, psychiatrists and GPs are all medically trained and are technically the only ones who are able to give you an official legal mental health diagnosis. That said, many therapists are familiar with the diagnostic criteria and will likely have a good idea of what is going on for you and how they can help. If an official diagnosis is required, they can write to your GP, outlining the symptoms and their concerns, and ask for assistance in referring you for a consultation with a psychiatrist or clinical psychologist who can make an official diagnosis.

Can I have more than one therapist?

Generally, this is not seen as a good idea as things could get confusing if each therapist were to take you in different directions. However, there are times when this can safely happen in practice; for example if you have couples therapy it will be done with a different person to who you have individual therapy with, and some work, for example EMDR therapy for trauma, requires a more specialised therapist.

Hiding things from your therapist

There can be a temptation to 'win' at therapy or to get it right, to be the best client, to frame everything in such a way that makes us look 'good'. Maybe even to the point where we don't let the therapist see the full picture and, therefore, we don't allow them to be as helpful as they could be. Or maybe we have deep trust issues and, although we might believe our therapist is safe, we still feel we can't share everything with them. We are simply turning up, keeping things light and on safe ground, talking about topics we know we can handle or even out-and-out lying to our therapist about what's going on.

I reckon most people will hide things from their therapist at one point or another, but a way to get past this is to understand more about why you might be doing so:

▶ You worry your therapist might judge you, but maybe it's actually something you're ashamed of yourself.

▶ It feels too embarrassing to talk about (particularly if it's something to do with sex, for example, and you don't feel you can talk to your therapist about such an intimate topic).

▶ You are in denial about the extent of the issue yourself.

▶ You've been betrayed in the past and find it really difficult to trust people.

▶ You worry your therapist might not believe you, especially if you've not been believed by people in the past.

▶ You are avoiding having to deal with something you know will likely cause you pain or shame.

▶ You are just not ready to talk about it yet, and that's OK – there is no set formula for healing.

One way some of the things I'm subconsciously hiding pop out is what my therapist and I call the 'door bomb'. This is where I divulge a whole session-worthy topic right at the end of the session, maybe even when I'm standing at the threshold of her door, that I should have brought up at the beginning.

The problem is, by dropping one of these what I'm really doing is avoiding the pain or discomfort that comes with discussing the difficult topic with my therapist because, let's be honest, a quick 30 seconds feels a whole lot easier than a full 50 minutes in the spotlight. But what I'm actually doing is just cheating myself out of getting the most out of therapy.

TALK ABOUT THERAPY IN THERAPY

It may sound a bit meta to talk about therapy in therapy, but it's something I'd recommend everyone does from time to time. For example, speaking up about the ways therapy is or *isn't* working for you is a really important part of the process. Maybe you feel your therapist is dedicating too much time to talking about your relationship and you don't feel that's productive for you. Or maybe you want your therapist to push back against your bullshit more. It might feel uncomfortable, but a good therapist will listen to your concerns and correct course, within reason.

BUT I JUST GOT STARTED

The feeling that your session is ending too abruptly is very common. It might be because you've just dropped a 'door bomb' or, more frequently for me, it tends to be because it's taken me some time to work through something, and just when I feel I'm getting to the good stuff I hear the soul-crushing words 'That's all we have time for today.' What feels like mere seconds later I'm left in a bewildered daze on my therapist's doorstep not quite knowing if I'm coming or going. It's hard not to feel frustrated and a little put out when this happens, but know that it's not because your therapist doesn't care – they just need to be firm with their own boundaries for your sake as well as theirs. I'd definitely recommend jotting down where you were and what you're thinking so the following week you can pick up more easily where you left off.

It can be hard to know when therapy is working for you and when it isn't because success in therapy is a pretty slippery concept to try to measure. Healing in therapy is very often non-linear, leading us to question at times whether we are doing it right.

It is important to note that 'doing it right' will vary from person to person, given that successful therapy for someone who has social anxiety is likely to look vastly different to someone who goes in order to increase their self-awareness or insights, for example. Then throw all various therapies, therapists and client goals (which of course could very well change and evolve over time) into the mix, and there really can be no standard metrics we can use to see whether we are getting it right or not.

That said, some therapists will use recognised tools or scales in order to monitor or measure your improvements, for example

♥ JO'S TOOLKIT: HOW TO SUPPORT SOMEONE ELSE AFTER THEIR THERAPY

▶ Give lots of extra TLC.

▶ Be available for them to talk to you, but don't demand or expect that they do. Respect their right to privacy if they don't feel like sharing.

▶ Try to remember it's about them and not you.

▶ Keep supporting their decision to get help. Therapy is hard, so keep being their cheerleader especially when it's tough for them.

▶ Understand they might be upset or exhausted afterwards. This is normal and doesn't mean there is reason for alarm.

▶ Be patient – therapy takes time, don't expect immediate results.

▶ Consider getting some support too.

the GAD-7 questionnaire, but many will not. However, there are things you could try yourself in order to track your progress. For example, if you are in therapy with certain behaviour-based issues, such as anxiety, you could keep a simple log monitoring whether your symptoms have generally increased or decreased over time. Trickier to measure would be the less tangible self-awareness improvements. For these, taking some time reflecting on whether you feel you understand yourself, feelings, motivations or behaviours a little bit more than before you started therapy might help. It's worth noting though that normal dips and plateaus don't mean therapy isn't working or you're not doing it right. Therapy doesn't mean you will never experience emotions like sadness and anger, or feel pain, but it should help you better cope and bounce back when they do come along.

Therapy thoughts

Natasha Devon MBE, mental health and body image campaigner and writer, tells me that she'd wished she'd known *'that when time's up, that's it. It's really disconcerting the first time you're pouring your heart out and your therapist is like "Right! That's the end of your session!" It feels really abrupt.'*

Chapter Twelve
OUTSIDE THE
Therapy Room

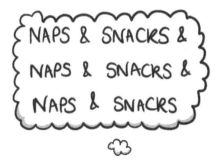

NAPS & SNACKS &
NAPS & SNACKS &
NAPS & SNACKS

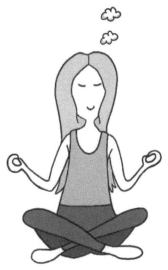

A hugely overlooked aspect to therapy isn't actually the time in the therapy room itself, but how we spend our time once we leave our therapist's office; how we think about and act on our therapy, and how we view therapy in our own lives. The importance of the time spent between each session, from the obvious acting on lessons recently learned, to the slower internal percolation of change that can passively play out over many years, sometimes long after our sessions have ceased, often gets underestimated and forgotten about.

How we carry our sessions away from the therapy room and into our real lives is how any real or lasting change happens. Because, putting it bluntly, at some point we need to get our butts off the proverbial couch and actually enact the techniques or lessons we have learned, make better or more conscious choices, or change the patterns that have held us back if we want to make change. This isn't magic; the therapist can't snap their fingers and magically all our problems will have disappeared. No, instead we need to put what we learn inside the therapy room into practice in our daily lives. A little like taking lessons to learn a new musical instrument, you pay for time with the instructor and then you go home and are expected to practise. When you return for your next lesson, if you've practised you hopefully will be better able to connect with what you learned last time and also with what you'll learn this time. If you don't practise between lessons, it doesn't mean you won't make any progress at all, it just might take longer, in some cases quite a lot longer, to build skills and make connections between new concepts.

As soon as you leave your therapist's office, whether it's to come back again next week or for the final time, my prediction is your therapist will be hoping you will incorporate the work you've just done into your daily life. Depending on what you're seeking therapy for, there will be any number of things that could help aid the work done in therapy. These could range from medication and support groups to alternative therapies. The ideas below offer some tips on how you can do productive work between your sessions that should help you to enhance, and more than likely accelerate, the work done inside of your sessions.

However, I want to stress that it is crucial to work at a pace that feels comfortable for you. These tips are only for those who feel able and comfortable in enhancing the work they are already doing inside therapy. It's perfectly OK for you to simply show up to your sessions without doing any active work in the interim.

HOMEWORK

Depending on the type of therapy you have, some might be a little more or a little less 'homework'-heavy and can range from the very concrete to the somewhat vague. A common example of a concrete piece of homework would be the exposure and response technique often used in OCD work. This is where you expose yourself to whatever it is that normally elicits a compulsive behaviour or reaction, for example you touch the light switch seven times before you go to bed, but you then do your best to refrain from that behaviour. And something more subtle might be for you to simply try to notice when you have a particular automatic thought or think about what you learned to make better sense of it, or maybe just for you to uncover new insights for your next appointment.

Being perfectly honest, I've found that I haven't particularly enjoyed or benefited from the more homework-heavy therapies. But this is probably more about the stage in my life I was at when I was trying to do them. For example, trying to do the CBT homework with a small baby felt far too overwhelming for me

– I wasn't prioritising myself and everyone else was coming first. At that time in my life, adding yet another spinning plate to the already precarious number that were up there, as well as wading through the sticky oppressive fog of depression, felt too much to take on. This is yet another reason why it's important to find not just the right therapist for you but also the right therapy (see Chapter Ten).

My current therapist has never set me homework, though the one before occasionally did, but chose to call it 'experiments'. And I have to say I prefer this term immeasurably. For some reason, being tasked with a little experiment doesn't bring the same heft of obligation as having to do my homework. It's funny what effect a tiny change in language can have, but it worked – I was far more willing to give her experiments a whirl.

One such experiment was conducted on a girl friendship group I had. There was a 'queen bee', as there so often is, and I was beginning to feel she might be directing a certain amount of passive-aggressiveness my way, which then the whole group would mirror. My therapist and I decided that I would try to just notice exactly when it was happening as it was often subtle and easily missed. I'd always leave the group feeling a bit rubbish about myself but not able to work out why, until the later dissection of what was said and how back in my therapist's office. Just trying to notice something in the moment might not sound very active, but my word did it work. Just this little experiment of bringing awareness to the situation was enormously powerful. Somehow by noticing it in the moment, it allowed me to take a tiny step back, unexpectedly cushioning and protecting me. It helped me to feel a little more in control, a little less emotional, a little less upset by the experience and ultimately, over time, it helped me feel able to change my relationship with this group for the better.

But let's be honest, no one really likes homework, do they?

Even the most studious among us will still have flashbacks to that heavy Sunday night feeling of something looming over our heads. If you find yourself dodging any work your therapist has set you, this little list of questions might help you to uncover why:

Are you putting everyone else first?

Once you've given to your partner, your children, your friends, your parents, your colleagues and your dog, you may struggle to find any remaining resources for yourself. As a mum (and dog owner) myself, this is something that I constantly struggle with. I know I need to prioritise my time for self-care and self-reflection, but, in the moment, it can often feel very counter to my natural instincts. It can feel as if there simply aren't enough hours in the day. If this is you too, I get it, it's hard. So hard. But when you do prioritise yourself, even just for a few moments each day or week, it can and does make a huge difference to not just you but everyone else around you too.

Do you have too high expectations?

As a perfectionist, I often set myself impossibly high standards in all areas of my life and suggestions made by my therapist are no different. And let's just say, if I don't get things right first time my motivation to try again can dip hugely. The shame and negative self-talk that come along with finding things tricky can also get in the way of giving new ideas and strategies a try.

What are you scared of?

It doesn't matter how much you may want it, change and uncertainty is unquestionably bloody scary. Not being able to predict what happens next can feel paralysing and often prevents us from moving forward. Adapting our outlook on the world, behaving differently in relationships and forgiving others and ourselves definitely hold transformational power. But it's really important to remember that you and your therapist should always proceed at a pace that is appropriate and comfortable for you.

Is change actually what you want?

Sometimes I have wondered whether we are all conditioned slightly too much by society to be constantly striving for change in our lives. Change is almost held up as the must-have Holy Grail, but what if we don't want to change? Ultimately you are in charge of how your life unfolds. You have the right to accept yourself as you are and live your life as you see fit. Sometimes, therapy will help you realise you don't want to or you aren't ready to change. You get to make that choice, no one else. Whatever you do, make sure your choice not to change is the one that feels right for you.

Is homework going to work for you?

Homework isn't the be-all and end-all. There have been so many times when I won't think about therapy between my sessions at all. Sometimes things are just too painful or heavy to keep in my conscious awareness, but I have found the next time I revisit the issue, I realise it has in fact been worked on in the background on a subconscious level. Or I'll notice that I've changed a behaviour without really thinking about it in any active way. So, if it feels like you're not doing anything, don't beat yourself up – taking things slowly and at your own pace is no bad thing.

JOURNALING

A lot of people find journaling a hugely helpful way to record their reactions to and reflections on their sessions, or things that come up during the week that they might want to raise in their next session. One person I know actually takes her journal into her sessions and has been known to read parts of it out loud to her therapist ,saying she often finds it difficult to articulate exactly what she's thinking and instead finds it easier to write it down. Journaling or note-making can also serve as a useful memory jogger if you find yourself not knowing what to talk about or drawing a total blank when you step inside your therapist's room.

RECORDING

I've never done this, but I do know some people who record (with the permission of their therapist of course) their sessions on their phones and then listen back in the week in between. I hate the sound of my own voice, so I'm not sure if I'd be comfortable listening back to my therapy waffle, but I can see how relistening could allow for ideas to sink in more deeply or be seen from a different angle, therefore enhancing what has been learned or said during the session.

READING

Many therapists will recommend books that might not only help heal you or help you grow, but also help you see that you aren't alone. My current therapist definitely likes to recommend books she thinks I might find helpful.

NON-THERAPY THERAPIES

No chapter about work done outside of the therapy room would be complete without talking about all the many wonderful and very therapeutic pursuits there are out there. I'll hold my hands up, it's not all that catchy, but I call these 'non-therapy therapies'. You know what I mean, things like meditation, yoga, being in nature, nights in, nights out, picnicking, pottery, painting, baking, breathing, running, dancing, cycling and horse riding.

We often hear people say when extolling the virtues of these activities, 'Oh, I don't need therapy, I have the gym, music, massage, my dog, crochet... etc.'. To this type of sentiment, I have a few things to say.

First, that's great. After all, there are many effective ways to let off steam, switch off or get more deeply in touch with how our bodies or minds work. Talking to friends, colleagues, religious or spiritual guides, family and teachers is a genuinely cathartic way to get things off our chests or find solutions to our problems. Equally, many of us gain a great deal from inward reflection through pursuits such as yoga, meditation, spirituality or religion in order to overcome challenges. For many people these activities will be more than enough to help them look after their emotional well-being and mental health, live in the moment and get in flow. However, for many others they will not.

Last year I challenged myself to try out a new 'non-therapy therapy' every day for the month of June (see the box below for my non-therapy therapy challenge ideas you might like to try out). Thirty days of jumping in and trying things out – from acupuncture to horse riding – and seeing what I liked and didn't. And the conclusion I came to? Well, they were are all wonderful ways to help me switch off and relax, save for crochet, which my mum tried to teach me but it didn't end well, but the less said about that probably the better. However, for me anyway, none could be conflated with therapy. Put simply, they are not therapy. They can be part of therapy sure, such as dance, art, play, music and drama therapy. But alone they just aren't therapy. Therapeutic, absolutely, but therapy, no. Therapy has unique characteristics that are very hard or impossible to find elsewhere, such as how trained and knowledgeable therapists are in helping people with their problems, or how your therapist's code of ethics and duty of confidentiality will help keep you safe, the sole focus on you and the uniquely one-way nature of the relationship.

Second, as I've said a number of times during this book, I truly believe not everyone *needs* therapy but pretty much everyone could *benefit* from it. Just because comfort, healing, growth and change can be found within other activities, it definitely doesn't mean you wouldn't or couldn't benefit from therapy as well. A great example of this is a friend of mine who, in her own words, 'used the gym as her therapy' when going through a difficult relationship, separation and eventual divorce. For a while this worked really well – the rush of endorphins, the sense of achievement, feeling and seeing her body getting stronger, and being part of a community all helped her enormously. But not so long ago she saw that she had been using the gym to keep the hurt away, bandaging the wounds, and sensed now was the time to stop avoiding it and get some help to dig deeper, fully move on and heal.

And finally, before I step down from my soap box, let's not forget it's not a case of being in one camp or the other. Without a shadow of a doubt, all these truly wonderful activities are yet further ways to enhance the work done inside the therapy room outside of each session.

MY NON-THERAPY THERAPY CHALLENGE IDEAS

1   Time with family and friends

2   Cinema/crap TV/box sets

3   Time off social media

4   God/church/spiritual time

5   Meditation/mindfulness

6   Breathing

7   Being in nature/outside

8   Mountain/coastal walks

9   Cuddles with pets

10   Sunshine

11   Picnic in the park

12   Breakfast outside

13   Gardening

14   Adult colouring/painting/art/drawing

15   Embroidery/sewing/knitting/crochet

16   Pottery

17   Long shower

18   A hot cup of tea

19   Exercise: the gym

20   Exercise: running/cycling/dancing

21   Yoga/Pilates

22   Cold-water swimming/swimming

23   Horse riding

24   Singing (in the car)/listening to music (loud)

25   Laughing

26   Bread making

27   Cooking

28   Silent time

29   Reading/listening to podcasts

30   Writing/journaling

WHEN THE TIME BETWEEN SESSIONS
FEELS TOO LONG: SELF-SUPPORT

Wrapped inside the safe cocoon of my therapist's office I can feel so secure and comforted; it's a place where I can release all of the pressure built up over the previous week. But on the outside of that protected space, back in the real world, life can sometimes feel a bit frightening, overwhelming and the pressure

BUMPING INTO YOUR THERAPIST IN THE PUB

True story, although it wasn't quite in the pub, more like outside of it. Me, a stumbling drunk uni student rather mortifyingly dressed as a schoolgirl, him my undoubtedly sober middle-aged psychiatrist stepping out of the cinema. I'm not sure who was more shocked than the other, although he did a manifestly better job of concealing it than my high-pitched squeal followed by my unsteady wobble away back into the safety of the pub.

To avoid my level of embarrassment, it might be a good idea to discuss running into each other with your therapist and have some ground rules for if this happens. Maybe you want to think about whether you're happy to be acknowledged by your therapist at all. Will you say a polite 'hello' and leave it at that? If your therapist is with someone else and they need to explain who you are, you might want to think about how they will introduce you, perhaps as a 'friend of a friend'? Or are you perfectly happy for them to say you are a client? All food for thought.

too much to bear for the seemingly never-ending stretch of time before I can return to my refuge of safety and release. So how can we keep as well as possible between visits, particularly if there is any kind of extended break?

In a bid to make this book as practical as possible I asked my current therapist whether she had any tips or suggestions to help people manage their symptoms or prevent their problems from developing or getting worse, particularly if they find themselves unable to access support for any period of time; for example they're on a waiting list, their therapist is away or they've decided to take a break from therapy for a while.

As she is certainly from the 'not-giving-advice' school of thought, she'd like me to stress these are merely suggestions and what works for one person might not be the answer for someone else. Also, it's important to acknowledge there is often only so much within our control and therefore there is only ever so much that we can do to change our circumstances. But having said that, the important thing to know is that there are very many things you can try that could help you, and the trick is to give them a go and find what works for you. And, better still, the tips listed below are all completely free.

Accept yourself

Sure, why not, let's start with a really big one! If you can crack this, it is definitely going to help you enormously in every area of your life. Don't beat yourself up if you don't master self-acceptance overnight though – it takes some serious hard work and effort to pull off.

Having self-acceptance means acknowledging and accepting that you are a complex, imperfect human being capable of making mistakes as well as significant accomplishments. It means accepting yourself in spite of your imperfections and because of your uniqueness. It also means you refrain from self-criticism, avoiding rating your self-worth based on what other people think, the way you look or when you perceive you do not live up to your own expectations. Research continues to show that self-acceptance is strongly related to mental health and well-being.

Be mindful

Practising mindfulness is a useful tool for everyone to harness. There are lots of different techniques, books and apps that will help you to do this. But essentially it involves making an effort to notice what is happening in the present moment (in your mind, your body and your surroundings) and accepting what's arising without judging it. It might sound counter-intuitive but being present and accepting what comes up without judgement can help you lower your stress and emotional pain. It can also help you increase your self-awareness (which, as we've seen above, is super important), manage unhelpful thoughts and develop more helpful responses to difficult feelings and events. And it really helps us see that we have more control over our thoughts than we might think. Again, be really gentle with yourself and keep your expectations low, especially when you are starting out. Mindfulness or meditation are tough and take a lot of practice at the best of times, let alone in the grip of a mental health issue.

Try controlled breathing

It sounds a little too good to be true, but scientific studies have shown that controlling your breath can help you to manage stress and stress-related conditions. By taking intentional deep breaths you can calm your emotional brain as well as your body.

There are a dizzying number of breathing techniques out there and it can be quite intimidating to know where to start or which technique is going to work for you. For me, as long as

I breathe out for longer than I breathe in, it seems to work its mood-boosting magic – with the added bonus that it's easy, free and you can do it anywhere from in front of your boss to on the bus!

Move your body

Physical activity has been proven to not only improve your physical health but also boost your mood, mental well-being, sleep and immune system.

It's important to add, though, that physical activity isn't always helpful for everyone's mental health. There might be times when you find it more helpful and others when it simply doesn't work for you. There are some people for whom physical activity might start to have a negative impact on their mental health, for example if you overtrain or have an eating issue.

Limit news and social media

While many of us enjoy social media, excessive use can fuel feelings of anxiety, depression, isolation and FOMO. It's important to remember that social media should never be a replacement for real-world human connection.

A recent study has found that reducing our social media use to 30 minutes a day results in a significant reduction in levels of anxiety, depression, loneliness, sleep problems and FOMO. But it also found that we don't actually need to cut back on our social media use that radically to improve our mental health; just being a little bit more mindful of it can have helpful results on our mood and focus.

Stay connected

Human beings are intrinsically social creatures. We need the companionship of others to thrive in life, and the strength of our connections has a huge impact on our mental health and happiness.

If the COVID-19 pandemic has taught us all anything, it's likely to be the importance of us staying connected even when we cannot physically be in the same room as others. Connecting with someone and talking about how you feel may sound like the last thing you want to do when you don't feel great, but being socially connected to others can ease anxiety, stress and depression, provide comfort and joy, boost self-worth, prevent loneliness, and even add years to your life.

Establish a routine

It might be one of the hardest things to do when you're not feeling great, but without a routine we can easily slip into feeling like we have no purpose, and with no purpose, we can find ourselves falling deeper into depression.

Try sitting down and writing out everything you do each day over the course of a week. Note if there is anything you can cut out or reduce and what other things you can give a set time to do each day or week. It's crucial that whatever you decide works with your lifestyle. If you like to stay up late, getting up early as part of your routine will probably not work.

Nail the basics

It might not sound particularly groundbreaking, but making sure we are eating properly, trying to get enough sleep and drinking enough water will all help us in the long run. That doesn't mean we need to pile any extra pressure on ourselves or feel guilty if we reach for the Ben & Jerry's once in a while or don't drink enough water in a day. But it will help our mood and well-being even if we are only a little bit more thoughtful and intentional about how we are treating our bodies and ourselves.

Surround yourself with a support team

This isn't always possible, but try to surround yourself with an understanding support team, whether that's supportive friends, family or colleagues. Feeling down or mentally unwell can feel incredibly isolating and lonely, making it even more important to have people in your life who either understand your condition or are willing to try.

Take it moment by moment

This little gem has helped me in so many ways in my life. I'm an overthinker, an over-worrier by nature, meaning I can end up stuck in paralysing spirals of panic or unhelpful thoughts. Forcing myself to focus on the present moment forces me to stop overthinking. You only have to google the term 'mindfulness' to discover that there are hundreds of different ways to achieve this, from gardening to guided meditations. But sometimes just simply reminding myself to take life one hour, or even half an hour, at a time, has in the past brought a lot of relief.

Be gentle with yourself

The term 'self-care' has been somewhat hijacked by big businesses and become synonymous with expensive spa retreats or bubble baths. My therapist uses the phrase 'be gentle with yourself', which I find far easier a concept to get on board with. It lands better somehow and allows me to stop punishing myself, stop pushing; it helps me to find relief, and caring ways to look after myself and relax. Somehow it gives me the permission I need to slow down, take things off my to-do list, celebrate the small wins, speak more kindly to myself, find time to relax or just 'be' without the guilt, and ease some of the constant pressure I put on myself.

Find out what makes you tick and do more of it! Find those

non-therapy therapies that work for you (see page 232). Don't know where to start? Maybe have a think about what you enjoyed as a kid and give it a whirl in your adult life. What tasks or experiences bring you comfort or relief?

Therapy thoughts

'While going to therapy is not always the easiest of choices, it is a decision that can have a lasting positive impact. Therapy is designed to be a safe space that invites authentic conversation and exploration without bias or judgement. Therapy provides perspective and support as one navigates life's challenges and makes the necessary room for healing to unfold. At the end of the day, therapy is cool because it is a standing invitation that one can accept at any point in life.'

Dr Christina Iglesia, licensed clinical psychologist and founder of the #therapyiscool mental health action campaign

Chapter Thirteen
WHEN THERAPY
Comes to an end

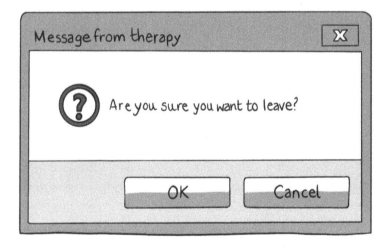

Message from therapy   X

(?)   Are you sure you want to leave?

OK   Cancel

All relationships, however long they last, will eventually come to an end somehow. And our relationships with our therapists are no different. Over the years I've learned that, as with any other relationship endings, particularly romantic relationships, these endings are often difficult but there are healthy and unhealthy ways to say goodbye.

That said, some of my less successful, shorter-term sessions have ended a little more neutrally, without much thought or emotion – brought to a close with curt professional nods, maybe a handshake, slightly uncomfortable but mainly very transactional in nature. But I should stress that these have been the exception rather than the norm.

The very nature of therapy means that it's personal and therefore the endings are nine times out of ten personal too. I've said it before and I'll say it again, yes it's a service relationship but it's akin to no other. Your dry cleaner isn't privy to how you really feel about your in-laws. Your landlord will probably never sit through a panic attack with you. Your local farmers' market person didn't help you build the self-support you needed to confront your boss.

Therapy is way more personal.

I'm ashamed to admit that I've definitely dumped a fair number of therapists over the years, most along the emotionally immature avoidance lines of 'It's not you, it's me'. 'See, I'm all better now,' I've proclaimed, 'I'm fixed, totally OK now, bye' and then bolted for the hills. One reasonably recent example when I knew after only a few short sessions it wasn't working out, I decided to start my next session with the words, 'This is going to be our last session with each other' before realising I had another 49 toe-curlingly embarrassing minutes to fill before I was free.

Then there's the therapist I ghosted entirely. I wince to think of it now, but one day I just didn't turn up. I refused to reply to their texts or emails, I hid my head in the sand and I never went back. I simply disappeared without so much as a backwards glance or a 'peace out'.

At that time, I hadn't understood something that seems glaringly obvious today: therapists are not automatons or robotic receptacles for other people's feelings. They aren't vending machines for empathy and positive regard. I'm sure when they get dumped, or ghosted, it hurts and they are left with a shed load of unanswered questions, like why, what went wrong, was it something they did to drive us out of the door, how long have we wanted to leave them for, what could they have done better, are we OK, did we get run over by a bus?

For me therapy is all about building an authentic relationship with a caring other and when that is broken, by either side, it is going to be tough to deal with. I can say this with good authority because the dumping doesn't just work one way. I was once abruptly 'terminated' – and yes that's the actual language that was used – by my psychiatrist while I was at uni. My depression was in full swing, meaning I'd carelessly missed two appointments in a row without realising. The consequence was severe – a letter informing me of my immediate discharge from his care and a very clear understanding that there were to be no second chances. It felt like I'd been floored by an actual physical blow. Our sessions were often stilted, and I don't think I ever really let him in, but still it felt like he'd cut off a much-needed lifeline. Something that was keeping me afloat somehow. I begged, I grovelled, I pleaded to be reinstated... which I eventually was, but things were never really the same between us again after that. Like when you're dumped by a partner, I think I couldn't put my ego aside to be able to get over the feeling of betrayal. And even though his reasons for cutting me loose were my own doing, I couldn't quite trust him again, and, as we have seen, trust is the cornerstone of a good therapeutic relationship.

♥ JO'S TOOLKIT: HOW TO BREAK UP WITH YOUR THERAPIST

1   *Talk to them first*. Instead of just ghosting, try bringing up the issues you're having to see if you can solve them without moving on to someone else. Say something like, 'My goals from therapy are XYZ and I'm concerned we're not meeting them together. What are your thoughts to help me get closer to achieve these goals?'

2   *Do it face to face*. Although it's scary, not only does it help give you both closure, it's a good challenge if you have trouble ending things or, like me, are a conflict-avoidant people-pleaser who hates feeling like you're upsetting someone. A therapist is probably the best type of person to practise on!

3   If after speaking to your therapist nothing changes or they don't seem receptive, it's totally OK to look for another therapist. Depending on the urgency of the issues you're working on, you might want

to lock in another therapist before quitting your current one. Although it's not usually advisable to have two therapists (see page 219), if it's on a short-term basis only it's likely not to be too much of an issue. Also, if you're actively dealing with a serious situation, like severe anxiety or depression, it's really important to have continuity of support.

4   Right, you've done all of the above, but how do you actually break up with them? Here are some suggestions on what to say:

▶ 'I think I've made a lot of progress in our time together, and I feel that now is the time for me to move on.'

▶ 'I want to end our work together because my goals have changed.'

▶ 'I've tried several sessions, but I don't think we are the best match.'

▶ 'I really appreciate your willingness to help me, but I realise I need something different now.'

▶ 'A few weeks ago, I mentioned [XYZ]. I don't see enough of a change for it to make sense that we continue together.'

In the end, remember that therapy is for you, so if you feel like you're not getting what you need, that's often more than reason enough to decide to end things. A good therapist will listen to what you feel is the best decision for you. And while they might disagree with you as they think you could benefit further, don't agree to continue if you truly wish to stop. They should be able to handle the break-up professionally and should not take your decision personally.

Saying goodbye to Elinor was sad and heartbreaking, but ultimately it was a healthy, or you could say a 'good', goodbye. I was moving away from London and I was clearly in denial about having to leave her. But I did eventually tell her, with a long enough lead time for us to have a good few months to talk it through.

And I am so glad that I did, because we explored our ending with the same curiosity and interest we did any other topic. Collaboratively we worked through all the many endings leaving a place I had lived and worked for many years brought, and how ending my relationship with her slotted into a phase of goodbyes in my life.

I hated the thought of leaving her, but I loved being able to have her support with finding a new therapist after my move. She helped me work through, with gentle compassion, my feelings of loss and grief at having to say goodbye to her as well as helping me to be able to reflect with her about how much I'd come to appreciate and find comfort in our time together. In a kind of bittersweet graduation, during our very last session she told me how much she enjoyed her Thursday mornings with me and how she was proud of what I'd achieved with her in the little garden office. Her words were the most precious goodbye gift she could have ever given me, and I suspect she knew their power and how I would keep them close to me for many years safely stored in the secret centre of my being.

DEPENDENCY

I think there is a difference between unhealthy and healthy dependency in therapy. When dependency is healthy we can rely on our therapists to provide a stable, healthy relationship to lean on in times of need as a source of empowerment, not a power drain. But a less healthy dependency is likely at play if we feel too paralysed to make our own life decisions without the input of our therapists. So, what do you do if you suspect you might be depending on your therapist too much? It might be awkward, but the main thing I'd suggest is to be honest with them if you think you might have become too dependent on them. Any therapist worth their salt will work on this with you to make sure the relationship is a healthy one.

In a strange way, I feel as if our 'good' goodbye sealed in the value of our sessions together, allowing me to carry them and the lessons learned in them for many years, rather than any good work done being tarnished by an awkward, rude, abrupt or uncomfortable goodbye.

SIGNS IT MIGHT BE TIME TO BREAK UP WITH YOUR THERAPIST

They don't get you
Seeing a therapist whose identity differs from yours in almost every conceivable way is not necessarily something that should

concern you. However, for many people the reason for being in therapy might be to discuss the very aspect of their identity that their therapist doesn't share, for example their culture or religion, and they will need their therapist to understand this and bring an extra level of understanding and sensitivity to such sessions.

If you feel that your therapist is somehow not valuing the knowledge that you have about your own culture and experiences, you should definitely bring it up with them. As we saw in Chapter Five, it can be enormously important for our therapists to understand our issues, culture or background. And while it doesn't mean they need to match our exact experiences, they do need to be able to understand what it is to be like us and, crucially, we need to trust that they understand our experiences.

You don't grow

Growth in therapy is very rarely instantaneous and will depend on a number of factors, such as what type of therapy you're having, how dedicated you are, how often you see your therapist, how skilled they are, what has brought you to therapy and the issues you are working through, but you really should be seeing some kind of change over time.

Everyone is different and will need different approaches, but recently I had a therapist who I didn't keep for very long as I felt like I wasn't growing. She would let me talk through things completely on my own without reacting, leaving me to flounder, and it meant I just went around in circles and never really got anywhere. This really didn't feel like the best approach for me. I realised I craved actionable discussion and collaboration in my therapy.

You feel shit more than you feel good

In a perfect world, every week we would all come away from our therapy sessions feeling like we've had our burdens lifted from us. However, in reality, as we've talked about previously, it is very normal to occasionally leave therapy feeling upset, exhausted, drained or ruffled from the emotions that have been stirred around – aka the 'therapy hangover' (see page 117).

These feelings are normal and are very different from feeling troubled every time (or nearly every time) you leave because your therapist isn't sensitive to your needs, isn't listening to you or isn't helping with this exact kind of uneasiness. If you find yourself routinely leaving your sessions feeling worse than when you arrived, this is a pretty big red flag that you should be stopping, switching or shaking things up.

The fear is that we will be truthful and they won't handle it well, but the chances are they absolutely will and, rather than distancing you, it will enhance your relationship and bring new avenues for you to explore together. After all, they are highly trained and skilled people. And if they don't deal with it properly, well it probably tells you quite a lot about their suitability to be your therapist.

You don't trust them

We've seen several times in this book that trust really is a key ingredient in the therapy process, as one of the main points of therapy is to be able to open up. In the past I've certainly hidden much of myself from various therapists and it nearly always created an ill-fitting dynamic and never led to real emotional growth. You too may be a little reluctant to be totally honest about the aspects of your life that feel difficult or shameful. That's why it's so important that your therapist creates a non-judgemental, safe space where you feel you can bring up these topics. If you can't, it's going to be impossible to work through them.

JO'S TOOLKIT: SOME TRUTHS YOU ARE ALLOWED TO SAY TO YOUR THERAPIST

▶ 'I disagree with that.'

▶ 'I don't feel like we fully addressed [ABC]. Can we go back to that?'

▶ 'I'm feeling really uncomfortable right now.'

▶ 'I feel you let me down.'

▶ 'I don't feel heard by you.'

▶ 'I don't feel like we are connecting on this'.

▶ 'I'm not ready to share that.'

▶ 'I don't think you understood me.'

▶ 'Could we move on from this?'

▶ 'Am I boring you?'

They are defensive

I had a therapist once who constantly started his sessions with me late, making me feel irrelevant to him, and then really rushed to get through everything in even less time, so one day I finally plucked up the courage and I told him how I felt. Instead of doing what a good therapist should do and taking the constructive criticism on board, he was angry and defensive, giving me a guilt-free pass to go and look for therapy elsewhere.

It's not practical

Therapy has got to work for you on a practical level not just an emotional one. Maybe you need evening appointments, but they don't do this or have none available, maybe you move, making it impractical to travel many miles a week, or they change office locations and don't offer any remote options. If you find yourself being unable to make or keep appointments, it might be time to see what else is out there that might work better for you.

You feel ready to leave

We don't always end therapy because it isn't working for us. Sometimes we will just know we are ready to stop. There might be less and less to say at each session, or perhaps we have increasingly found the solutions to any issues that have popped up in between our therapy sessions and we feel our initial goals have been met. Ideally, we'd all only ever be leaving because we are happy with the outcomes and ready to move on with our lives without therapeutic support. If you start feeling you've learned everything you can from your therapist, it could be a good time to start discussing leaving.

WHAT IF I'M NOT READY?

It can be tricky to know exactly when to leave therapy as life often presents new challenges that therapy can invariably help us with. Perhaps our goals have shifted, and we continue to want support with our new ones.

Something else to consider is whether thoughts of ending things with our therapist coincide with an elephant in the room we don't want to address. Is there something we are avoiding talking about and we think the therapist might actually be getting a little too close to our vulnerable truth? And maybe we might think it would be easier to end our therapy than face our reluctance or the uncomfortable issue head-on.

Sometimes the end of therapy is something we have little choice over. Perhaps one party is moving away, maybe the therapist is retiring or cutting their workload, our insurance sessions may have ended or our allotted free NHS sessions have run their course. Whatever the reason, therapy ending before we are ready can be the cause of regret, frustration and anger. You might feel disappointed, abandoned, cross or helpless. These are all very normal reactions you should discuss with your therapist to see if they can help you work through them.

If there is a relocation involved, for you or your therapist, you might explore telephone or online sessions, either in the short term while you find another therapist, which is what I did with Elinor, or it might even work out as a more permanent longer-term solution. If they are cutting their workload, retiring or leaving they might be able to refer you to someone else they recommend and think you would suit, and while shifting to a different therapist might feel overwhelming and disruptive, it might actually be an unexpected chance to find new insight and growth with someone different.

TO HUG OR NOT TO HUG?

It's a big regret of mine that I didn't ask Elinor for a hug on our last session together. If I'm honest, I was afraid of the rejection if she said no. I didn't want our goodbye to be tarnished by me overstepping the therapeutic boundary.

But what I'd say to anyone else pondering this is it's absolutely OK to ask for a hug. Every therapist will be different; some might be relaxed about it and others might have a strict no touching policy, with the possible exception of a handshake. Whatever their policy, they should explain their reasons for wanting to maintain the boundary of no touching or why it might be OK in a particular circumstance.

In terms of insurance sessions ending, again it is worth talking to your therapist about this. They might be able to offer you a lower fee going forward or recommend services that provide more affordable options or sliding scale fees based on what you can afford. For more about lower cost options see page 201.

The short-term therapy provided for free by the NHS is brilliant as it gives much-needed support for many. However, on the flip side, time-limited support and a severe lack of funding in a struggling system mean often you wait for months on a waiting list, to then only barely scratch the surface and, before you know it, you're back trying to deal with things on your own. Just as you get going, as it often takes a few sessions to settle in and open up (more about the first session in Chapter Eleven), before you know it you're screeching to an abrupt halt. Long-buried issues are stirred up, only for you to be unceremoniously dumped and left to try to come to terms with them without the ongoing support. As an aside, I have it on good authority that in most parts of the country you will be able to re-refer yourself for further support under your local IAPT service; some areas will put a cap on the number of times you can do this for the same issue, but others won't. However, each referral would mean another stint on a waiting list.

Sadly, without a huge injection of government funding, there is currently no obvious solution if you find yourself in this situation, since our health system in the UK is struggling, and unfortunately it is extremely short of resources and professionals. Take a look at Chapter Ten as there might be other free or low-cost options available to you.

CAN I COME BACK?

Returning to therapy, whether with the same or a different therapist, is something that is very much a possibility. I have a friend who sees her therapist roughly once every six months, like little therapy top-ups, and then opts for more regular sessions if she feels the need. And as mentioned above, you may be able to self-refer multiple times under your local NHS IAPT service.

That said, there can be a feeling that if we return to therapy we have failed somehow. A feeling of we haven't been able to cut it on our own or we've regressed or relapsed in some way. And while this could be true in some cases, very often it won't be, particularly if therapy has helped us on previous occasions. It is more likely we now know therapy is a positive influence and a helpful way to support us with a new challenge.

Therapy thoughts

Elinor tells me, 'Therapy is a collaboration between therapist and client. The therapist's job is to create a space where the client feels heard and where the client can feel able to disagree with something. If you don't feel comfortable, speak up. Or find another therapist.'

FINAL WORD

Hopefully this book has shown you all the wonderful ways therapy really is magic... for me. And my hope is that you too will experience some of the magical wonder of therapy.

But of course, it is important to recognise that therapy will be different things for different people and it won't hold the same magical properties for all. The great thing about therapy is that you're not required to go. If you don't like it, no worries; you don't have to go back. If you only want to go once a month, that's great too. Or if you just want to go once to see what it's like, you can totally do that too. Therapy is all about what works for you, and only you. And truly that's probably the most magical part about it.

Therapy has been a huge part of my life. I have experienced first-hand how powerful and life-changing it can be to have someone there beside you, supporting and encouraging you while you navigate the hard stuff. I have felt the magical transformational power of being heard, being listened to, being accepted and being valued.

It feels really quite special to be able to share with you as the book draws to a close that, during the course of writing this book, I have started my own psychotherapy training in order to one day be able to share the magic of therapy in a different and much more personal way with my own clients. It feels like the most fitting way to give back some of the magic I've experienced, to be able to accompany another human on their journey of self-discovery and change, to go full circle in my own journey with therapy and at the same time be able to shine some magical light into another person's life. Surely that is the best job of all.

Therapy really is magic.

Jo Love

RESOURCES

CRISIS SUPPORT
Help and support is available right now if you need it. You do not have to struggle with difficult feelings alone.

In an emergency
Call 999 or go to your local A&E department.
If you're in crisis and need to speak to someone
Call NHS 111 (for when you need help but are not in immediate danger).
Contact your GP and ask for an emergency appointment.
Contact the Samaritans: 116 123.
Use the 'Shout' crisis text line: text SHOUT to 85258.

CHARITIES
Anxiety UK
For those affected by anxiety, stress and anxiety-based depression.
www.anxietyuk.org.uk

Bipolar UK
Empowers individuals and families affected by bipolar.
www.bipolaruk.org.uk

Black, African and Asian Therapy Network (BAATN)
Ensures people of Black, African, South Asian, Caribbean and People of Colour have the resources through which they can psychologically liberate themselves and live their lives more fully according to their ideals.
www.baatn.org.uk

Black Minds Matter
Provides free 12-week courses of therapy to Black individuals in the UK.
www.blackmindsmatteruk.com

Campaign Against Living Miserably (CALM)
A leading movement against suicide.
www.thecalmzone.net

Chasing the Stigma
Aims to remove unnecessary stigmas attached to mental illness and provides the database 'Hub of Hope', which sets out mental health services near you.

www.chasingthestigma.co.uk
www.hubofhope.co.uk

Cry-Sis
The only UK charity offering
help and support to parents with
babies who cry excessively or have
sleeping problems, they
offer advice as well as providing
a helpline to parents.
www.cry-sis.org.uk/

Maytree
Provides a unique residential
service for people in suicidal crisis.
www.maytree.org.uk

Men's Health Forum
Supports men's health in England,
Wales and Scotland.
www.menshealthforum.org.uk

Mental Health Foundation
Aims to find and address the
sources of mental health problems
so that people and communities
can thrive.
www.mentalhealth.org.uk

Mental Health Matters
Provides mental health support
services, ranging from helplines
and talking therapies to supported
housing and safe havens.
www.mhm.org.uk

Mind
Provides advice and support to
empower anyone experiencing a
mental health problem.
www.mind.org.uk

No Panic
Helps and supports those living
with panic attacks, phobias,
obsessive compulsive disorders
and other related anxiety
disorders.
www.nopanic.org.uk

OCD Action
Provides support and information
to anybody affected by OCD.
www.ocdaction.org.uk

OCD UK
Provides advice, information
and support services for those
affected by OCD.
www.ocduk.org

Pandas
A national PND awareness and
support mental health charity
offering a range of support to
parents, families and carers.
www.pandasfoundation.org.uk

PAPYRUS
Dedicated to the prevention of
young suicide.
www.papyrus-uk.org

Relate
The UK's largest provider of
relationship support.
www.relate.org.uk

Rethink Mental Illness
Works to transform the lives of
everyone severely affected by
mental illness, and how our nation
approaches mental illness.
www.rethink.org

Samaritans
Confidential support, whatever you're going through.
www.samaritans.org

SANE
Works to improve the quality of life for anyone affected by mental illness.
www.sane.org.uk

Switchboard
A one-stop listening service for LGBT+ people.
www.switchboard.lgbt

YoungMinds
Fighting for children and young people's mental health.
www.youngminds.org.uk

BEREAVEMENT SUPPORT
Cruse Bereavement Care
www.cruse.org.uk

Marie Curie
www.mariecurie.org.uk

BIRTH TRAUMA
AIMS Ireland
www.aimsireland.ie

Birthrights
www.birthrights.org.uk

Birth Trauma Association
www.birthtraumaassociation.org.uk

Make Birth Better
www.makebirthbetter.org

FINDING A THERAPIST
There are several directories that can help you find the right counsellor or therapist for you. Some of the main professional bodies also have directories.

Counselling Directory
www.counselling-directory.org.uk

Cultureminds Therapy
www.culturemindstherapy.com

Free Psychotherapy Network
www.freepsychotherapynetwork.com

Harley Therapy
www.harleytherapy.com

Improving Access to Psychological Therapies (IAPT)
www.nhs.uk/service-search/find-a-psychological-therapies-service

Pink Therapy
www.pinktherapy.com

UK PROFESSIONAL BODIES
Association for Cognitive Analytic Therapy Ltd (ACAT)
www.acat.me.uk

Association for Dance Movement Psychotherapy UK (ADMP UK)
www.admp.org.uk

Association of Child Psychotherapists (ACP)
www.childpsychotherapy.org.uk

Association of Christian Counsellors (ACC)
www.acc-uk.org

British Association for Behavioural and Cognitive Psychotherapies (BABCP)
www.babcp.com

British Association for Counselling and Psychotherapy (BACP)
www.bacp.co.uk

British Association of Play Therapists (BAPT)
www.bapt.info

British Psychoanalytic Council (BPC)
www.bpc.org.uk

British Psychodrama Association (BPA)
www.psychodrama.org.uk

British Psychological Society (BPS)
www.bps.org.uk

British Psychotherapy Foundation (BPF)
www.britishpsychotherapy foundation.org.uk
College of Sexual and Relationship Therapists (COSRT)
www.cosrt.org.uk

Counselling & Psychotherapy in Scotland (COSCA)
www.cosca.org.uk

EMDR Association UK (EMDR UK)
www.emdrassociation.org.uk

European Association for Gestalt Therapy (EAGT)
www.eagt.org

Federation of Drug & Alcohol Professionals (FDAP)
www.smmgp-fdap.org.uk

Health & Care Professions Council (HCPC)
www.hcpc-uk.org

Human Givens Institute (HGI)
www.hgi.org.uk

Irish Association for Counselling and Psychotherapy (IACP)
www.iacp.ie

National Counselling Society (NCS)
www.nationalcounsellingsociety. org

Play Therapy UK (PTUK)
www.playtherapy.org.uk

UK Association for Humanistic Psychology Practitioners (UKAHPP)
www.ahpp.org.uk

UK Association for Transactional Analysis (UKATA)
www.uka4ta.co.uk

UK Council for Psychotherapy (UKCP)
www.psychotherapy.org.uk

Universities Psychotherapy & Counselling Association (UPCA)
www.upca.org.uk

BOOKS

This is by no means an exhaustive list, but these are some of the books that have helped me:

▶ *A Beginner's Guide to Being Mental: An A–Z by Natasha Devon*

▶ *A Manual for Being Human by Dr Soph*

▶ *A Toolkit for Modern Life: 53 Ways to Look After Your Mind by Dr Emma Hepburn*

▶ *Anxious Man: Notes on a Life Lived Nervously by Josh Roberts*

▶ *Depression in a Digital Age: The Highs and Lows of Perfectionism by Fiona Thomas*

▶ *Hope Through Recovery: Your Guide to Moving Forward When in Recovery by Hope Virgo*

▶ *How Not to Be Good: The A to Z of Anxiety by Elli Johnson*

▶ *Know Your Worth: How to Build Your Self-Esteem, Grow In Confidence and Worry Less About What People Think by Anna Mathur*

▶ *Languages of Loss: A Psychotherapist's Journey through Grief by Sasha Bates*

▶ *No Such Thing As Normal: What My Mental Illness Has Taught Me About Mental Wellness by Bryony Gordon*

▶ *The Body Keeps The Score: Mind, Brain and Body in the Transformation of Trauma by Bessel van der Kolk*

▶ *The Book of Hope: 101 Voices on Overcoming Adversity by Jonny Benjamin and Britt Pflüger*

▶ *The Mind Medic: Your 5 Senses Guide to Leading a Calmer, Happier Life by Dr Sarah Vohra*

▶ *The Stranger on the Bridge: My Journey from Suicidal Despair to Hope by Jonny Benjamin*

▶ *Why Birth Trauma Matters by Dr Emma Svanberg*

NOTES

Chapter One: Therapy is Uncomfortable

James, S. L., Abate, D., Abate, K. H., Abay, S. M., Abbafati, C., Abbasi, N., & Briggs, A. M. (2018). Global, regional, and national incidence, prevalence, and years lived with disability for 354 diseases and injuries for 195 countries and territories, 1990–2017: A systematic analysis for the Global Burden of Disease Study 2017. *The Lancet, 392*(10159), 1789–858.

Chapter Two: Therapy is Awkward

Meier, A., & Boivin, M. (2011). The gestalt empty-chair and two-chair techniques. In: Meier, A., & Boivin, M. (2011). *Counselling and Therapy Techniques: Theory & Practice*. SAGE Publications, 46–60.

Chapter Three: Therapy is Overwhelming

MBRRACE-UK (Nov. 2019). Saving lives, improving mothers' care.

Chapter Five: Therapy is a Privilege

Goldsmith, S. K., Pellmar, T. C., Kleinman, A. M., & Bunney, W. E. (2002). *Reducing Suicide: A National Imperative*. National Academies Press, chap. 9.

Independent Review of the Mental Health Act 1983 (Dec. 2018). Modernising the Mental Health Act: Increasing choice, reducing compulsion.

Mental Health Taskforce to the NHS in England (Feb. 2016). The five year forward view for mental health. Retrieved from https://www.england.nhs.uk/wp-content/uploads/2016/02/Mental-Health-Taskforce-FYFV-final.pdf (accessed 7 Jan. 2021).

MIND (Nov. 2013). We still need to talk: A report on access to talking therapies.

Sturm, R., & Sherbourne, C. D. (2001). Are barriers to mental health and substance abuse care still rising? *The Journal of Behavioral Health Services & Research, 28*(1), 81–8.

Sussman, L. K., Robins, L. N., & Earls, F. (1987). Treatment-seeking for depression by black and white Americans. *Social Science & Medicine, 24*(3), 187–96.

The Tavistock and Portman NHS Foundation Trust (n.d.). Tavistock adult depression study (TADS). Retrieved from https://tavistockandportman.nhs.uk/research-and-innovation/our-research/research-projects/tavistock-adult-depression-study-tads/ (accessed 7 Jan. 2021).

Chapter Eight: Therapy is Magic

Cozolino, L. (2010). *The Neuroscience of Psychotherapy: Healing the Social Brain (Norton Series on Interpersonal Neurobiology).* WW Norton & Company.

Cozolino, L. (2016). *Why Therapy Works: Using Our Minds to Change Our Brains (Norton Series on Interpersonal Neurobiology).* WW Norton & Company.

Duncan, B. L., Miller, S. D., Wampold, B. E., & Hubble, M. A. (2010). *The Heart and Soul of Change: Delivering What Works In Therapy.* American Psychological Association.

Goldfried, M. R. (2013). What should we expect from psychotherapy? *Clinical Psychology Review, 33*(7), 862–69.

Ivey, A. E., D'Andrea, M. J., & Ivey, M. B. (2011). *Theories of Counseling and Psychotherapy: A Multicultural Perspective: A Multicultural Perspective.* Sage Publications, chap. 2.

Jones-Smith, E. (2015). *Theories of Counseling and Psychotherapy: An Integrative Approach.* Sage Publications, chap. 20.

Lambert, M. J. (1992). Implications of outcome research for psychotherapy integration. In Norcross, J. C., & Goldfried, M. R. (Eds.) (2005). *Handbook of Psychotherapy Integration.* Oxford University Press, 94–129.

Lambert, M. J., & Barley, D. E. (2001). Research summary on the therapeutic relationship and psychotherapy outcome. *Psychotherapy: Theory, Research, Practice, Training, 38*(4), 357–61.

Lambert, M. J., Garfield, S. L., & Bergin, A. E. (2004). *Handbook of Psychotherapy and Behavior Change.* John Wiley & Sons.

Lambert, M. L., & Vermeersch, D. A. (2002). Effectiveness of psychotherapy. In: Hersen, M. E., & Sledge, W. E. (2002). *Encyclopedia of Psychotherapy*. Academic Press, vol. 2, 709.

Malhotra, S., & Sahoo, S. (2017). Rebuilding the brain with psychotherapy. *Indian Journal of Psychiatry*, 59(4), 411.

Stamoulos, C., Trepanier, L., Bourkas, S., Bradley, S., Stelmaszczyk, K., Schwartzman, D., & Drapeau, M. (2016). Psychologists' perceptions of the importance of common factors in psychotherapy for successful treatment outcomes. *Journal of Psychotherapy Integration*, 26(3), 300–17.

Chapter Nine: Is Therapy For You?

National Institute for Health and Care Excellence (Oct. 2009). Depression in adults: recognition and management (clinical guideline [CG90]). Retrieved from https://www.nice.org.uk/guidance/cg90/ifp/chapter/treatments-for-mild-to-moderate-depression#psychological-treatments-for-depression (accessed 7 Jan. 2021).

Wang, P. S., Berglund, P. A., Olfson, M., & Kessler, R. C. (2004). Delays in initial treatment contact after first onset of a mental disorder. *Health Services Research*, 39(2), 393–416.

Chapter Ten: How to Find the Right Therapy for You

Mearns, D., Thorne, B., & McLeod, J. (2013). *Person-centred Counselling in Action* [fourth edition]. Sage Publications.

NHS (Mar. 2020). The improving access to psychological therapies manual. Retrieved from: https://www.england.nhs.uk/wp-content/uploads/2020/05/iapt-manual-v4.pdf (accessed 7 Jan. 2021).

Chapter Twelve: Outside the Therapy Room

Chamberlain, J. M., & Haaga, D. A. (2001). Unconditional self-acceptance and responses to negative feedback. *Journal of Rational-Emotive and Cognitive-Behavior Therapy*, 19(3), 177–89.

Fox, K. R. (1999). The influence of physical activity on mental well-being. *Public Health Nutrition*, 2(3a), 411–18.

Hunt, M. G., Marx, R., Lipson, C., & Young, J. (2018). No more FOMO: Limiting social media decreases loneliness and depression. *Journal of Social and Clinical Psychology*, 37(10), 751–68.

Zaccaro, A., Piarulli, A., Laurino, M., Garbella, E., Menicucci, D., Neri, B., & Gemignani, A. (2018). How breath-control can change your life: A systematic review on psycho-physiological correlates of slow breathing. *Frontiers in Human Neuroscience, 12*, 353.

ACKNOWLEDGEMENTS

I'd like to start by thanking my amazing agent Jo, who has believed in me, encouraged me and guided me so calmly throughout this entire process, even when this book was only a mere glint of an idea. Thank you to Lauren, my commissioning editor, for having faith and confidence in the book right from the off. To my fabulous editor, Julia, thank you for your patience, incredible craft and grace. I honestly couldn't have done this without you.

Thank you to all the marvellous contributors to this book who have been so generous with their time and words. Thank you also to the very many other professionals who have patiently explained concepts and processes, fact-checked and allowed me to pick their brains behind the scenes. Thank you for letting me interrupt your far-too-busy schedules.

To the man who told me I couldn't write. You will never read this because for you this book shouldn't exist, but without your impact on my life, it probably never would.

An enormous thank you to my wonderful friend Fiona who so magnanimously took up position as my 'unofficial book mentor', fielding unsociable voice notes, panicked WhatsApp messages and phone calls at all times of the day and night. Thank you Mills for your unwavering support and positivity, from sitting drinking wine on my kitchen floor surrounded by a million Post-it notes thrashing out the structure of this book, to allowing my book to become a part of your already incredibly busy life.

Thank you to my husband Chris for allowing me to share part

of our story here and unquestionably supporting this wild ride I have been on throughout what has been a chaotic time in our lives. Your unflappability and steadfast support have kept me propped up when I've needed it the most. Thank you for reading each chapter multiple times as I worked my way through, and thank you for pretending you liked doing it!

Thank you to my current therapist Kate, not only for gifting me your words, but for patiently being there for me week after week during this whole process. You've been there for the highs and the lows, you've allowed me to air my ideas and my frustrations, your support has meant the world to me and as such I feel this book is just as much yours as it is mine.

And to Elinor, thank you for showing me the real magic of therapy. Thank you for everything; without you this book really wouldn't have happened.

Last but not least, thank you Bella, I am forever grateful to you and your love.

INDEX

Dear Boo,

You've just turned five and you're skipping around the kitchen as I type, singing and dancing so joyously, lost in your own little world in the way that you do, making it so hard to imagine you being all grown and reading this.

Thank you for putting up with me. I'm sorry I didn't smile as much as I'd like, particularly in those early days. But please know your smiles and giggles bring me joy every day. Your laugh lights up my soul.

Thank you for all you have taught me. You might not know it yet, but you have brought the most amazing lessons into my life. As your mummy (and 'the Boss'), I might appear to know everything, but I want you to know, I don't. I'm still learning, every day and every moment. Our relationship is a two-way street and, as you will see, I'll give you as much knowledge as I can, but please don't ever stop teaching me.

Thank you for giving me such strong direction. Before you, I was just plodding along in life, mostly trying to please others. You have given me the motivation and determination to follow my dreams. You have brought meaning to my life and given me a direction. I'd be lost without you.

Thank you for being so determined. If it wasn't for your determination to get what you wanted, I would have been quite clueless. There were times when you cried a lot and were difficult to settle, but that's only because you were trying so hard to communicate what you needed to me.

Thank you for all the insights you have given me. I would never have seen the world as I see it today without you. I am truly grateful for that and I will pass on to you what I can.

Thank you for being you. I promise I will always do the best I can by you. Daddy and I will always be here for you for all of our days.

Finally, thank you for always being you. I adore you. You are wonderful.

I love you (a penny chew, a plastic whistle and a pot of glue),

Mummy x

ABOUT THE AUTHOR

Jo Love is a trainee psychotherapist, mental health advocate and artist.

Jo regularly speaks, writes, hosts events, workshops and talks on mental health. She shares her experience of mental illness including depression, anxiety and burnout alongside evidence-based strategies that helped her recover. She is a mental health ambassador for various brands and organisations. Jo regularly consults with companies, brands and schools on how to look after our mental health and help break the stigma that still sadly surrounds getting support.

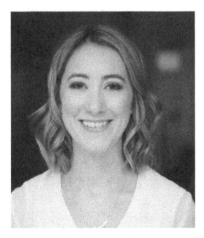

Nancy H Gibbs Photography

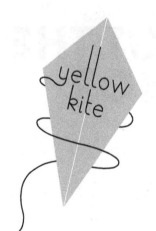

books to help you live a good life

Join the conversation and tell
us how you live a #goodlife

🐦 @yellowkitebooks
📘 YellowKiteBooks
📌 Yellow Kite Books
📷 YellowKiteBooks